Nature Cure & Health Care

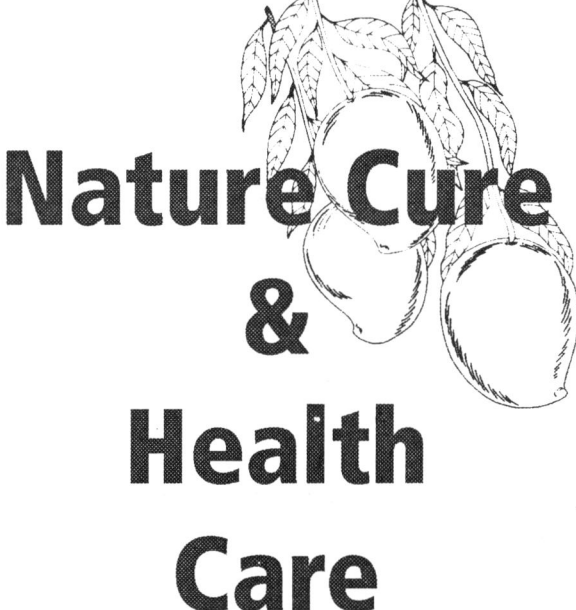

Binodini Debi

Edited by
Dr. Bhagbanprakash

HEALTH ＆ HARMONY

An imprint of
B. Jain Publishers (P) Ltd.
An ISO 9001 : 2000 Certified Company
USA — EUROPE — INDIA

NOTE FROM THE PUBLISHERS

Any information given in this book is not intended to be taken as a replacement for medical advice. Any person with a condition requiring medical attention should consult a qualified practitioner or therapeutist.

NATURE CURE & HEALTH CARE

Second Edition: 2003
Reprint Edition: 2005, 2007

All rights are reserved. No part of this book may be reproduced, stored in a retrieval system or transmitted, in any form or by any means, mechanical, photocopying, recording or otherwise, without any prior written permission of the publishers.

© Copyright with the Publishers

Published by Kuldeep Jain for

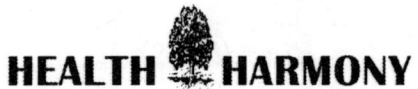

HEALTH HARMONY

1921, Street No. 10, Chuna Mandi, Paharganj,
New Delhi 110 055 (INDIA)
Ph.: 23583100, 23581300, 23581100, 23580800,
Fax: 011-23580471,
Email: bjain@vsnl.com
Website: www.bjainbooks.com

Printed in India by
J.J. OFFSET PRINTERS
522, FIE, Patpar Ganj, Delhi-110092

BOOK CODE:/ ISBN 978-81-319-0082-6

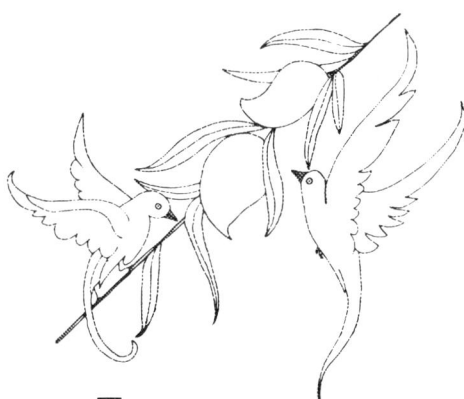

To Dr. Heera Lal, Mahatma Gandhi's close desciple, at whose feet we learnt the basic principles and practice of nature cure and health care.

"Nature cures, not the physician."

Hippocrates

CONTENTS

Nature Cure & Health Care ii
Preface v
Acknowledgement xi

PART I PRINCIPLES AND METHODS

Introduction 3
Our Body 5
Nature Cure: Brief History 7
Other Systems Of Treatment 9
    AYURVEDA 9
    UNANI 10
    ALLOPATHY 10
    HOMOEOPATHY 10
    REIKI 11
    MAGNETO THERAPY 12
Main Principles of Naturopathy 13
Basic Nature Cure Methods 15
    SOME NATURE CURE METHODS 16
    WATER CURE 18
    EARTH CURE 21
    AIR CURE 21
    FIRE AND HEAT CURE 22
    JUICE CURE 23

FASTING: THE FIRST MEDICINE 25
TOUCH THERAPY: MASSAGE 27
COLOURS AS SUPPORT THERAPY 30
ACUPRESSURE 31

PART II FOODS AND FITNESS

Living Foods: The Natural Medicine 37
High-Fibre Foods: Nature's Scavengers 41
Sprouts: The Wonder Food 45
Nature's: Superstars 49
Facts on Fats and Cholesterol 61
White and Sweet Poisons 65
Flesh Foods: Myth and Reality 69
Leaf Lovers and Cancer Fighters 75
Calorie: The Energy Tonic 79
Food Friends 83
    TYPES OF FOODS 84
    THE SPICES OF LIFE 85
Nature Diet from Nature Farm 89
Fitness for Freedom 93
Eating Plan and Detox Diet 97
Yoga: Healing Mind and Body 101
    KRIYAS 103
    ASANAS 104
    MEDITATION 111
Positive Thinking 113

PART III NATURE CURES

Common Nature Cure Chart for Good Health 119
Some Common Disorders and Natural Remedies 123
    RHEUMATOLOGICAL DISORDERS 123

RESPIRATORY DISORDERS 128
GASTRO-INTESTINAL DISORDERS 133
LIVER DISORDERS 139
URINARY DISORDERS 141
ANORECTAL DISORDERS 144
DIABETES 146
OBESITY 147
HIGH BLOOD PRESSURE 148
HEART DISORDERS 150
STROKES 152
CANCER 153
PYORRHOEA AND TOOTHACHE 155
HEADACHE AND MIGRAINE 157
INSOMNIA 158
DEMENTIA 160
MENSTRUAL DISORDERS 161
FEVER 162

Art of Natural Living: Basic Rules to Remember 165
Further Readings 169

PREFACE

There is a growing realization around the world that going away from Nature is in fact running away from good health. While 'back to nature' is good as a health message, the real challenge lies in its practice – as there is always a big gap between knowledge and behavior, between awareness and action, between attitude and practice.

THIS BOOK is more than a self-help or a do-it-yourself, everyday guide. It tries to familiarize the readers with the whole range of holistic healthcare and alternative therapies, skills and practices in which *Naturopathy* plays a pivotal role. The book shows how simple and inexpensive lifestyle changes could safeguard against a plethora of health problems caused by hectic and stressful modern-day living.

The high cost of medication and hospital services, and increasing rate of drug reaction have already rendered the doctor-medicine-hospital-treatment syndrome unsustainable and unfriendly. This has led to a rediscovery of the virtues of nature food, nutrition, exercise and positive habits as well as thinking. For instance, for obsessive compulsive disorders a form of talk-treatment called cognitive-behavior therapy or interpersonal-therapy is now found to be more effective than medicines. Similarly concepts like aroma therapy, color therapy, gem therapy, juice therapy and touch therapy are now being increasingly discussed in the world of alternative medicines. People's faith in these as alternatives to drugs and surgery is growing stronger. Consequently, more and more people are moving away from institutional medical care to individualized self-help and self-reliance.

In fact, many people are now looking at their own habits more closely. Vegetarianism, which used to be considered a food fad, has now earned new respectability and glamour as a healthy food habit. It is no longer confined to India or a few individuals in other countries. In UK alone, the number of vegetarians has doubled in just ten years. According to the UK Vegetarian Society, three and half million Britons are now its devotees and the vegetarian food market is worth £398 million a year. 'Love for the leaf', 'Romance with radish', 'Affairs with amla', 'Never say no to neem', 'Jogging for joy',' Fat to fit', are some of the slogans through which health magazines popularize the natural way of eating and living habits. Almost every day, well researched and scientifically documented facts and findings on various aspects of health foods are trickling in.

For example, a recent Harvard study of 48,000 women and men has found how exercise can cut the risk of colon cancer by half. Another four-year long study of 3,123 persons in the Netherlands has shown that those who consumed at least one onion a day had half the risk of suffering from stomach cancer as onion contains strong anti-cancer compounds.

Eating of brassica vegetables like broccoli, turnip, cabbage and cauliflower reduces such risks by 40 percent. Daily intake of 12 glasses of water and liquids reduces the risk by 32 per cent. Phytoestrogens in soya have very strong prostate and breast cancer fighting properties. Fibre, roughage and protective chemicals in fruits and vegetables rid the body of toxins and carcinogens and boost its immunity against diseases.

Recently researchers at the University of Illinois have confirmed something which naturopaths knew all along that honey is healthier than sugar and dark honey is healthier than light honey. The Illinois value-added Research Programme has also revealed that a daily garlic supplement could help prevent hardening of arteries that carry blood to the heart. The National Cancer Institute (NCI) in USA has now identified a number of anti-cancer herbs—onion, garlic, mint, basil, turmeric, ginger, coriander, cumin, aniseeds and parsley, which are regularly used in South Asian kitchen.

The genetic engineers are now working overtime to promote the primordial naturopathic concept of food as medicine. For instance, the New Zealand Institute of Crop and Food Research is now developing the concept of bio-pharming using vegetables and agricultural crops for large scale production of pharmaceuticals. The roof top Solarium of Singapore Polytechnic is turning the humble potato into a potential phamacentical factory producing low-cost vegetarian drugs for people afflicted with high blood pressure, kidney problems and congestive heart failure. Very soon such vegetable medicines are going to occupy pride of place in the shelfs of medical stores.

Recently, a trio of American (John B. Fenn), Japanese (Koichi Tanaka) and Swiss (Kurt Wuethrich) scientists have been awarded Nobel Prize (2002) for their outstanding contributions to a new science called 'proteomics', which studies how proteins, the stuff of life, could be developed into a new generation of food-based super medicines. Food hygiene is now considered as an answer to many fatal and incurable diseases. The study of human genome now has opened up immense possibilities of controlling diseases through food chemistry and diet modification.

Such findings only reinforce our belief in nature's powerful healing capacity and the importance of personal health decisions and choices.

As more people are readying to recognize health as a personal responsibility, the concept of healthcare has also undergone a change. Health is no longer considered as absence of disease, but a condition in which the body, mind and emotions are in harmony.

Since preventive is always better than the curative, the book emphasizes the need for a change in personal habits, health behavior and practices. It offers a holistic health abstract full of choices, options and alternatives which are simple, accessible, and practical. As most of the health problems in middle and old age are the result of faulty lifestyles during the youth and early adult years, the book continuously reminds the readers about the benefits of a balanced living which is supported by hard facts and well researched scientific data.

The book also aims at demystifying healthcare, and bringing it within the control of an individual. It gives authentic information to the readers about the value of food as medicine. The chapters and sub-chapters on air, water, fire, earth and color therapies provide valuable insights along with new information on vegetarianism, and flesh foods and the '27 superstars of nature'.

The drugless Common Nature Cure Chart (CNCC) with which the treatment section begins, is by itself a very dependable guide to healthy living. The tips on positive thinking as an integral part of natural living may be of special significance to the reader.

The author has tried her best to give as much information as possible on Naturopathy. The book combines conventional healthcare wisdom, practical experience and principles of Naturopathy in a lucid, reader friendly presentation.

The book also tries to convince the readers that Naturopathy is not an ethnic or occult system of treatment based on beliefs and assumptions, but is rooted in sound scientific judgments, and now corroborated by epidemiological studies as well as research findings. ■

Dr. Bhagbanprakash

ACKNOWLEDGEMENT

- Respected Dr. Heeralal. You are no more and yet you are always in my mind when I prescribe nature cure tips and emphasize the value of uncooked food.

- Dr. A.P. Dewanjee. You used to quote Hippocrates, who said: "Illnesses can only be treated by nutrition." I always follow this mantra.

- Prof. (Dr.) Vinod Mishrajee. I shall always remember your encouragement and deep commitment to Naturopathy despite being a Professor of Aviation Medicine.

- Dr. N.S. Adhikari. How can I forget you! Your tireless zeal and dedication for the cause of Naturopathy is exemplary.

- Bipin Bhai. You revealed to me the secrets of acupressure to relieve pain and suffering of people.

- Dr. Kasinath Panda and Dr. Usha Jain. I learnt from you the simple ways of drugless cures.

- Through my association with all of you, I realized that the best doctors in the world are—Doctor Diet, Doctor Quiet and Doctor Merry. I take this opportunity to thank you all for your goodwill and best wishes.

- Dear Readers. Please don't forget that your health is in your hands, and that real health can be found beyond doctor, medicine and hospital. This book is an attempt towards that end. Don't follow it blindly take professional advice—as each human body is unique.

- Thank you Manoj, Gayatri, Maitri and Prakriti for all your encouragement and cooperation. A special thanks to Pradeep Nayak for assisting with preliminary layout, typesetting and artwork.

- My husband, friend and guide, Dr. Bhagbanprakash, continuously inspired me to put down my ideas and experiences in the form of a book and undertook the strenuous task of writing the preface, polishing, editing and improving the text with his insights. Thank you for realizing my long cherished desire. ∎

Author

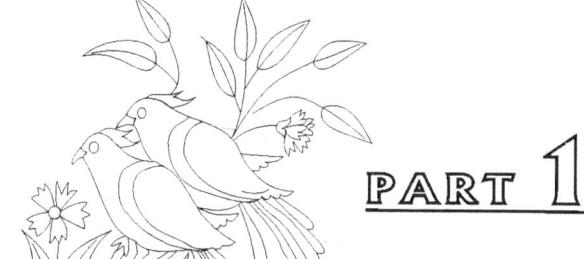

PART 1

PRINCIPLES & METHODS

"Pure food promotes pure mind and pure mind develops life and memory."

Manu Smriti

INTRODUCTION

About two thousand years ago, Hippocrates, now called as father of Modern medicine, referred to the "Vis medicatrix Natural" — the healing power of nature.

IN FACT, Nature, through a long process of evolution, has prepared and programmed the human body to live at least for 120 years. However, our changing lifestyles, eating and living habits, and environment continuously interfere with this natural lifespan and expose the body and mind to various influences.

Health and diseases are two conditions of the same body. But there are endless interconnections between the two. Medical literature offers numerous definitions of these two conditions. According to the World Health Organization (WHO): "Health is a condition of complete physical, spiritual and social well-being and not merely the absence of disease or physical defects." This holistic definition recognizes the ecological relationship between the internal and the external living conditions of women and men. Humans and nature have developed critical interdependence during the process of evolution.

It is a known fact that the living cell with its complex biological structure and metabolic processes has been existing in nature for more than three billion years. While the most ancient ancestor of Homo Sapiens, Ramapithecus, lived eight million years ago, the present humans as we know them, evolved about forty thousand years ago. It is believed that the Australopithecus (southern ape) lived about 2.6 million years ago and began walking erect on two feet in response to changing conditions of the environment including landscape and climate. Thus, environment became the natural medium in which Homo Sapiens and their body evolved slowly.

The five major components *(Panch Mahabhut)* of the environment are the *sky, air, fire, water* and *earth*. Naturally, the physical body is a microcosm made of these five major elements. The oxygen surrounding us, the solar rays and the water on land formed the basis of creation out of which human beings also originated. Thus, these elements became an integral part of life, activities and survival of the human organism.

The principles and practice of Naturopathy are based on these facts and factors. It looks at women and men as children of nature. Their health and happiness is influenced by nature. It treats their diseases through rational use of natural healing agents like earth, air, water and sun. *In this way, Naturopathy is a drugless, harmless, holistic therapy that promotes healing and health by reinforcing the self-curative forces within the body.* Thus, a Naturopath is not a doctor and does not treat or cure, but helps and guides through a natural way of living by self-control, diet management, yoga, exercise and positive thinking. In that sense naturopathy is in fact, a superpathy based on the basic principle that all healing comes from within the body. The body can cure itself. ■

OUR BODY

HUMAN BODY has been created by nature through a long process of evolution extending over a few million years. The principles of naturopathy can be applied to human body effectively only after proper understanding of its structure, functions and relationships of its constituent parts to one another. First of all, one has to understand the Regional Anatomy, a physical study of arms, legs, head, chest etc. followed by a study of bones, muscles, nerves, blood vessels and so on known as "Systemic anatomy". The study of relationships between parts and structures of the body is also important which are grouped under functional anatomy allied to the study of physiology. We find many parts of the body are symmetrically arranged like right and left eyes etc. But there is also a good deal of asymmetry i.e. spleen on the left side, liver on the right side and pancreas on both the sides.

The body is also divided into various systems arranged according to their functions. So we have Locomotor System concerned with the movement of the body, Circulatory System that transports blood, Digestive System that breaks down food by enzymes, Respiratory System that manages breathing by taking oxygen from the air and breaths out carbon dioxide, Urogenital System that expels waste products and functions as sex and reproductive work.

Then there are special sense organs like taste, smell, light, hearing and testicle functions of the skin. The body is also made up of tissues and organs. The smallest unit of this is the cell that reveals the complex chemistry of life.

Human body is supported by a framework called skeleton. It provides support and protection for some soft organs and acts as levers in movement of the body. The skeleton is also full of joints surrounded by muscles and covered by skin.

A good naturopath must have a thorough understanding of the human anatomy and physiology of both female and male as naturopathy emphasizes on drugless cures by reviving the inner strength of the body beautiful. ∎

NATURE CURE
BRIEF HISTORY

Nature cure treatment is very ancient and was in practice in Egypt, Greece, Rome, India and China.

THE PRINCIPLES of *Panch Mahabhut* or five elements of nature were practiced in India as an effective means of treatment for various diseases as far back in time as 2500 BC. *Yoga* and *Pranayama* were essential parts of this process. Although Hippocrates (460-357 BC), the father of modern medicine, had advocated methods of nature cure in the West, the modern methods of nature cure originated in Germany in 1822 when Vincent Priessnitz established the first *water cure centre* there. However, it was Dr. Benedict Lust (1872-1945) who developed various successful natural experiments as a system of treatment called Naturopathy. Therefore, he is known as the father of naturopathy. As it grew popular, students of naturopathy developed various methods creating a vast body of knowledge and skills on the subject.

Naturopathy became popular in India when Mahatma Gandhi adopted and advocated its usefulness. Soon thereafter, the number of followers and admirers continued to rise. Today, there is a network of nature-cure and yoga centres all over the world drawing a large number of followers. ■

OTHER SYSTEMS OF TREATMENT

AYURVEDA

THERE ARE several systems of treatment. The system closest to the principles of Naturopathy is *Ayurveda* (Science of Life) which originated in the Vedic period and developed from various Vedic hymns which described the essentials of nature, life, disease and treatment.

Around 1000 BC, the Ayurvedic treatment was systematically recorded by *Charak* and *Sushruta,* two renowned Indian physicians. This healing system is based on the theory that all living and non-living beings in the world are made of *'Pancha Mahabhutas'* i.e., earth, water, fire, air and the sky.

The physiological entity (or the humour) of a living being is determined by the combination of these five elements. The human body is a combination of three *humours* or *Tridosha* (air, bile and phlegm), seven body tissues, five senses, mind, intellect and soul.

According to *Ayurveda*, a person is healthy when all these constituents coexist in a structural and functional state of equilibrium.

UNANI

Another popular treatment system is *Unani*. This system originated in Greece during 460-377 BC, and came to India with the Arabs and Persians. It is based on the theory of humours stating that there are four such humours in the body, namely, blood, phlegm, yellow bile and black bile. These are reflected in temperaments—sanguine, melancholic, phlegmatic and choleric respectively. The system aims at re-establishing the original humoural constitution of the individual. It makes use of plants, minerals and animal products as curative agents, and tries to activate the self-preservative mechanism of the body.

ALLOPATHY

Allopathy is a very widely practiced system of treatment which originated in the West. It is based on the biomechanical concept of life and tries to correct physical or mental illness with medicine or surgery. Its emphasis is on symptomatic relief. In the field of communicable diseases and surgery, allopathy is far more advanced compared to any other system of treatment.

HOMOEOPATHY

Homoeopathy is another system of treatment which believes in the principle, *'Similia Similibus Curantur'* (Let likes be treated by likes it can produce). This unique principle was discovered by Dr. Christen Frederic Samuel Hahnemann, a German physician. Like Ayurveda and Unani, this system also lays emphasis on strengthening the immune system of the individual.

While all these systems make use of drugs, Naturopathy is a

drugless treatment. It applies simple laws of nature to cure diseases by modifying eating and living habits and adoption of purificatory measures.

REIKI

Rediscovered by Dr. Mikao Usui, in Japan and the U.S.A.

This age-old healing practice called REIKI is becoming increasingly popular as a spiritual healing process. It is an art of healing and cure by means of placing the hands on the body of the patient. Originally formulated by Buddhist Sages of India, China and Tibet. Reiki is derived from the Japanese word "Ray-Key". "Rei" or "Ray" means universal and "Ki" or "Key" is the life force energy or spirit. Reiki in practice is very akin to Yoga that attempts to unite body and mind. Like Yoga, Reiki claims to be independent of religion belief or faith systems. In Reiki healing the energy flow comes from the spiritual source via a pillar of light that connects the individual to spiritual through crown chakra, third eye chakra, throat chakra, collecting in heart chakra flowing down further to the hands and wherever hands are placed. Reiki energy is believed to flow directly to the chakras and from there to the endocrine system that produces hormones – helping a balance of health. The recipient of Reiki undertakes to follow five principles in life in order to get results of the treatment. These are:

1. Just for today – I will not get angry.
2. Just for today – I will not worry.
3. Just for today – I will earn a living honestly and decently.
4. Just for today – I will be grateful and give thanks for all the blessings in life.

5. Just for today – I will show love and respect for every creature and every form of life.

MAGNETO THERAPY

In this healing system, the ailments are treated by application of magnets to the body of the patient. Although the healing properties of the magnet were known to the ancients, it reemerged as a therapy in the 16th century. The use of magnet as a healing agent is mentioned in Atharvaveda. Mother earth itself is a huge natural magnet and its magnetic field can be detected to a distance of 1,05,600 kilometers from its surface. In this therapy magnets work in the body to regulate blood circulation, nervous, respiratory and other natural systems of the body. The human body is basically made up of tiny cells which are also tiny magnets. Magneto therapy claims to be rooted in natural law and treats patients by facilitating an interplay between magnetic fields in the body and outside. ∎

MAIN PRINCIPLES OF NATUROPATHY

"A Doctor's smile can often heal more than two weeks of antibiotics."

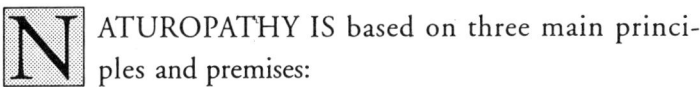ATUROPATHY IS based on three main principles and premises:

(i) According to Naturopathy, it is not the germs but morbid matter in the body that causes disease. These waste materials pile up steadily through years of faulty habits and wrong lifestyles. Therefore, all nature-cure methods first enable the body to throw out these morbid matters.

(ii) The second basic premise is that all chronic diseases are the consequences of continued suppression of acute diseases through drugs and vaccines.

(iii) The third premise is based on the fact that the body has an inherent power to heal itself if right methods and positive habits are adopted, not drugs or doctors. When drugs are used, the patient has to recover twice—once from the illness and once from the reaction of drugs. So, for our health problems nature is the medicine, nature is the doctor and nature is the hospital. ■

BASIC NATURE CURE METHODS

WHILE MODERN medical methods tend to treat each symptom and disease as a separate entity, Naturopathy *treats the organism as a whole and tries to cure a disease by stimulating and reviving the inner vitality of the body.* It looks at each individual as a unique personality with her or his own body chemistry, biological clock, rhythm, genetic code and hormonal system. This unique system is exposed daily to various external influences. Food plays a critical role in this process. So, as a *first step* the patient is advised to *regulate the diet* to get rid of the toxins accumulated on account of wrong and *irregular eating habits.* Acid forming foods like proteins, starches and fats are excluded for a week, and replaced with a fresh fruit diet. The stomach and alimentary canal are thus *disinfected.*

If the system is overloaded with morbid matter and toxins, a complete juice and water fast for days is prescribed with regular enema every morning.

Depending on the nature of the disease, *massage, hip bath, mud-pack, throat pack, stomach pack, gastro-hepatic pack, steam bath, sun bath, yoga* and *deep breathing* are recommended. These are further reinforced by a high residue and high fibre, well-balanced diet, with plenty of green vegetables, pure drinking water, fresh air, regular exercise and clean hygienic habits.

SOME NATURE CURE METHODS

(Indicated briefly; to be followed in consultation with a qualified Naturopath).

Hip Bath

1. Can be given cold, hot, neutral or alternate.
2. Level of water should cover hips up to navel.
3. Rub abdomen softly for 15 minutes.
4. After such bath—jog, walk or do yoga.
5. During hot bath (40 degree centigrade) drink a glass of water and apply cold compress on head.
6. *Variation:* Hot for 5 minutes, cold for 5 minutes then hot, and ending with cold.

Spinal Bath

Spinal bath, like hip bath, can be given in cold, hot or neutral temperature. The water in tub should cover the entire length of the spine from the nape of the neck. Duration is 15 minutes. Constant water temperature is to be maintained.

Hot and Cold Compress

1. Two small pieces of towel—one piece to be soaked in warm water and wrung out.

2. Keep on abdomen for 3 minutes—hot water bag can be kept on it to maintain temperature.
3. To be followed by towel soaked and wrung in cold water and placed on abdomen for one minute.
4. Process to be repeated 3 times.

Hot Foot Bath

1. Place cold compress on head and drink one glass of water.
2. Dip both legs in a bucket or tub filled with hot water (40 degree centigrade).
3. Cover body with a blanket.
4. Duration 15 minutes—temperature to be maintained by adding hot water.
5. Cold shower may be taken after this.

Packs

1. Can be used for chest, throat, kidney, liver, abdomen and girdle.
2. For kidney, place hot water bag to cover space between chest bone and stomach; wrap or softly tie a cotton cloth and flannel over this for 45 minutes.
3. Gastro-Hepatic pack can be given covering the liver and abdomen.
4. For chest pack, dip cotton cloth or small towel in cold water, wring out, place on chest and cover it with dry cloth for 45 minutes.
5. For throat, wrap cold cloth around the neck with a dry cloth on top and dry flannel on it for one hour.

6. For girdle pack, dip underwear in cold water, wring out water and wear. Cover with thick, dry cloth for 45 minutes.

7. For mud packs, place cleaned soaked mud on a muslin cloth and place on abdomen for 25 minutes. Pack length—10", breadth—6", thickness—1".

Enema

1. One litre of pure warm water with juice of one lemon or a glass of boiled *Neem* water.

2. Smear enema *nozzle* with oil or Vaseline for easy insertion.

3. Lie on the right, insert nozzle in the rectum and pump in the water.

4. Retain for 5-10 minutes. Remember to remove air from the tube by letting some water flow out before insertion.

Fomentation

Water temperature may be 40-45°C. Either hot water bag or cotton cloth can be used. When hot water bag is used, area of application may be covered with cotton cloth wrung in cold water.

Steam Inhalation

Water is heated till steam is generated. Inhale the steam through nose by covering the head with towel. Duration is 7-10 minutes.

WATER CURE

Nature has provided all the five elements with great curative properties. Among these, water has been used for centuries to cleanse and soothe the body. Ancient Greeks, Egyptians, Hebrews, Japanese, Persians, Indians and Chinese used water as a remedy. Centuries before Christ, Hippocrates used hot and cold water for fever, ulcers, bleeding and joint pain. *More than sixty percent of our body weight is water.* Muscle tissues contain 75 percent of water. Even in case of bones, water content is 22 percent. Many of the fruits and vegetables we eat are full of water. About 84 percent of an apple is water and 78 percent of a Potato is water. Each one of the 100 trillion cells in the body is filled and bathed with it. We can not live more than a few days without water. It is the basis of all body fluids. Water is also an extremely important nutrient and *fundamental to health and fitness.* It checks the viscosity (thickness) of the blood, equalizes circulation, aids digestion and nutrition, tones up activity of the respiratory gland, eliminates damaged cells and flushes out toxin from the body.

It is a fluid replacer as well as natural diuretic and is central to various metabolisms. It cleans out both the kidneys and the bowels. A teaspoonful each of honey and lemon juice in 2-3 glasses of lukewarm water in the morning is one of the best *health tonics* against chronic constipation and many other diseases. On an average, we need one glass of water for every 200 calories we expend. For 2500 calories a day to keep the body moving, one needs at least 12 glasses of water.

Recent research has *scientifically established the healing value of water.* Diseases like headache, hypertension, obesity, arthritis, diabetes, rheumatism, sinusitis, bronchitis, asthma, acidity, constipation, dysentery, urological problems and menstrual disorders can be cured by water therapy. Five glasses of pure water in the morning in 15 minutes cleans the system thoroughly and forms new and fresh blood. No food or beverage should be taken after it for 45 minutes. The effect of this practice can be felt in two days.

Water is a *miracle fluid.* It cradles the body, relaxes and caresses it with force of waves, backwash and fluid resistance. It gives an unique freedom and flexibility to the body. That is why swimming is considered one of the best exercises. In water, muscles can be stretched and extended and joints are mobilized without strain.

Water therapy, a free gift of nature, is becoming popular. Athletes exercise in water pools for Olympics, pregnant women attend aquatic classes, elderly people, the handicapped and the injured are cured by water based physiotherapy. All one needs for water or hydrotherapy is a bucket and a basin or bath tub at home and a large jug on the desk, always full of pure drinking water for the day.

The other important use of water is in washing. We cannot think of basic hygiene without water. The most expensive soap or detergent is useless without water. It is water which *can wash off millions of germs and bacteria from our body.* Even an ordinary bath in clean water refreshes a tired, aching body. Cool water bath creates an invigorating effect. Tepid water bath gives a relaxing, soporific feeling. Warm water bath takes away aches from a tired body.

The other therapeutic uses of water are enema, cold compress, hot compress, cold and hot hip baths, spinal bath, full wet sheet pack, hot foot baths, steam bath, etc. Mineral and hot water or sulphur springs have cured more diseases than modern medicines.

EARTH CURE

Naturopaths lay great stress on the curative properties of earth. Application of *pure clay* acts as a natural bandage for wounds and injuries. Sleeping or lying on earth vitalizes the body. *Walking barefoot on grass in the morning gives energy and strength to the system.* Mud packs and mud baths are two popular methods in nature cure for successful treatment of a number of diseases. For a variety of ailments, sprains, boils and wounds, fever, measles, kidney or liver disorders, rheumatism, chronic inflammations, a mud pack is highly effective.

The wetness in the mud pack opens the pores of the skin, draws blood to the surface, relieves tumour constriction and pain, promotes heat radiation and eliminates morbid matter.

For *preparing mud pack,* clay is collected 10 cm below the ground level. *The clay should not have impurities, composts or pebbles.* The clay is then made into a smooth paste in warm water, and after cooling, spread on a piece of cloth. The pack is applied on abdomen or other parts of the body according to the nature of ailments for 10-30 minutes.

Mud or clay bath is another form of treatment. It is prepared in the same way as mud pack but is applied all over the body. It has a great curative effect on various types of skin disorders. It relieves pain in the joints and other parts of the body. The duration of mud bath is normally 30 minutes to one hour after which the body should be cleaned with warm water.

AIR CURE

The body can live without food for long days, and without

water for a few days, cannot survive without air and space for even five minutes. We go on inhaling and exhaling air continuously and indefinitely. The air we inhale is known as *prana* or life force. The system of *Pranayam* is based on this. Fresh, open air is an important factor for health. It imparts strength and vitality to the body. Like water or mud bath, air bath is life-giving. Walking in the shade or greenery with white loose cotton for half an hour in the morning does a world of good to the body. Deep breathing and air bath strengthen and freshen all the nerve endings in the skin and improve blood circulation.

Similarly our body is also composed of molecules and atoms. Each atom is 99.9999 percent empty space. The subatomic particles moving at lightening speed through this space are actually bundles of vibrating energy. This energy break down further into an empty void. And this void in the body vibrates with unseen intelligence inside the DNA. This flow of intelligence is the real Prana, the life force that sustains all of us.

FIRE AND HEAT CURE

This element is manifest through the sun, the source of all power. It gives energy to plants as well as animals. It prepares and processes food in the plants for our use. It gives colour to the skin and vigour to the body. Human body gets vitamin D mainly from the sun through the skin. Infra red rays of the sun benefit the circulatory system and the muscle. Adequate sunlight is needed for the growth of bones and prevention of rinklets. Like air bath, sun bath increases immunity of the body. The best period for such bath is in the morning hours *when the sun is young*. But remaining in the sun for long hours is detrimental to health. It destroys the elastic fibres that are responsible for youthful appearance.

While sunbathing one should always have the back towards the sun and take a glass of water before and after the sun bath. The heat generated by fire or sunlight opens up blood vessels in the skin. Oxygen in superficial capillaries increases and blood gets diluted with more plasma. Red blood cells increase.

Steam baths and hot fomentation have a beneficial effect on joints. Hot compress relieves pain. Hot baths reduce abdominal pain, flatulence, spasm of colon, muscles and joints. Hot spring baths eliminate skin problems, rheumatoid arthritis and dermatitis.

JUICE CURE

Fruit, root and vegetable juices are considered very effective *food-medicines* provided by nature. Full of vital enzymes, nutrients, organic chemicals and trace elements, juices serve as the tonic of life. Most fruit juices are absorbed by the system within fifteen minutes. As the enzymes in the juices are pre-digested, they provide *instant energy* to the body. That is why, a fast should always be broken with a glass of fruit juice.

Fruit juice is also a great cleanser. It purifies the blood, expels accumulated toxins from the cells and revitalizes the body. On the other hand, vegetable juices are *prime generators* and help in many chronic diseases, strengthen the nerves, promote glandular activity and, most importantly, restore *acid-alkaline balance* in the body.

Broadly juices are divided into six types:

(i) Juice from sweet fruits like custard apple and grapes;

(ii) Sub-acid fruits like apples;

(iii) Acid fruits like orange;

(iv) Vegetable fruits like tomato, cucumber.

(v) Green, leafy vegetables like cabbage and spinach, and

(vi) Root vegetables like carrot, beet root, potato, radish etc.

Juice therapy needs proper planning. Two liters of juice mixed with a litre of pure water taken one glass full at two hourly intervals every day helps the patients expel toxins and regenerate the system. For this, the right kind of fruits, root or vegetables are to be selected as each and every fruit or vegetable has its own unique blend of vitamins and minerals.

For instance, orange offers vitamin C, fibre and folic acid. Lemon and lime are powerful anti-oxidants with cancer fighting and anti-ageing properties. Juices from dark fruits like grapes, cherry and berries are beneficial to people with low blood pressure, heart and kidney problems. *Amla* juice is highly beneficial to people with liver problems and low blood sugar. Apple juice contains cancer fighting anthrocyanins, fights high cholesterol and prevents colon cancer. Tomato juice, high in carotenoid lycopene, lowers the risk of prostate cancer. Mango juice contains vitamin B6 essential for healthy blood.

Juices from lentils stave off high blood pressure. Bitter gourd juice destroys disease-causing bacteria and viruses and is very effective in diabetes. Cabbage and carrot juice are very effective in cleansing the intestines and help in controlling anemia, liver troubles, acidosis, blood poisoning, circulatory disorders, ulcers, gall stones and gout.

Juice of pineapple and grape enhances immunity. Wheat grass juice is a known fighter against blood cancer. Spinach juice furnishes vital missing nutrients in the roots of the hair and has a great anti-clogging effect, guarding against heart disease. Citrus juice therapy is effective for cough and cold.

Sugarcane, beet and radish juices are quick healers of jaundice, hepatitis and other liver diseases. Grapes, spinach, lettuce and beet root juices are of great help in correcting menstrual disorders. Cucumber and papaya juice help control constipation and colitis. Arthritis is treated with juices from sour cherry, sour apple, cucumber, lemon and carrot. Lemon, grape fruit, cabbage and lettuce juice are very useful in treating obesity.

Withdrawal from juice therapy should be gradual. To begin with, it should be replaced by milk and fruit and then by a light balanced diet. Juice therapy can be continued for four weeks without any problem under the expert guidance of a naturopath. However, it is imperative that the patient is able to take adequate rest during this period to consolidate the benefits from the therapy.

FASTING: THE FIRST MEDICINE

In Naturopathy, fasting is observed as a *method of self-purification*. It is also practiced in many religions. Muslims, Sikhs, Hindus, Jains, Buddhists and Christians, all observe fasting as spiritual practice. It is nature's most effective and *least expensive medicine* for treatment. Charak, Susruta, Hippocrates, Galen, Paracelsus and many great authorities on medicine have regarded it as a very dependable and curative method. It is a common knowledge that even when animals and birds fall ill, they withdraw from food, and therefore, recover faster. A recent 14-year study (AP, Philadelphia) has found that dogs who ate less lived nearly two years longer and developed fewer chronic diseases than those allowed to eat as much as they wanted.

The modern lifestyle, irregular eating habits, overeating and consumption of junk food, repeated use of drugs, sedentary living and lack of exercise generate lot of toxins and morbid matters in the body. These impurities affect the digestive and assimilative organs. They derange the system and clog the internal cleansing process.

As an unclean drain spreads infection, an impure organism invites diseases. Fasting, by depriving the body of food for some time *helps the bowels, kidney, lungs, and liver expel disease-causing toxins and impurities.* Additionally, it gives the needed rest to critical organs in the body. According to Dr. Ranger Berg, an international authority on nutrition: "During fasting, the body burns up and excretes huge amount of accumulated wastes."

Types and Methods of Fasting

There are three types of fasts:

(i) Water fast;

(ii) Juice fast; and

(iii) Mono-diet fast.

Traditionally, pure water fast was practiced but fasting on juice is considered more beneficial. For certain diseases mono or single fruit or vegetable diet like bitter gourd, papaya, wheat grass juice, grapes, cucumber, etc., is prescribed because of their curative properties. *Fasting on alkaline juice* eliminates uric and other inorganic acids. Vitamins, minerals, enzymes and trace elements in fresh fruit and vegetable juices restore body's balance and revive its vitality.

The juice should be diluted in pure water and one glass should be taken very 2-3 hours. *During fasting, enema should be taken every alternate day.* The total liquid intake should not be less than 10-12 glassfuls in a day. *Physical rest and mental relaxation* is essential during fasting. Simple exercises like short walks may be taken followed by a *lukewarm water bath in the morning.*

To start with, fasting may be done once in a week or a fortnight for a day or two. For certain chronic or critical diseases the duration varies from one to four weeks under strict guidance of a qualified naturopath. Breaking of fast must be gradual with a light and liquid diet for 1 or 2 days before resuming the normal diet. *Over-eating after fasting* defeats the very purpose of fasting.

Benefits

During fasting the body decomposes, burns and destroys diseased cells and tissues. The eliminative organs like lungs, liver, kidney and skin are revitalized. Accumulated wastes and toxins and expelled. The process of digestion is improved. The *body engine is overhauled, cleansed, serviced and fine-tuned.* Fasting, dieting and moderate exercises bring about rapid reduction in weight of the obese people. Long-term fasts should be under proper guidance.

TOUCH THERAPY: MASSAGE

A natural way of reviving the body is the healing power of touch. We instinctively touch our forehead, temples, eyebrow when we feel tired or pained. Touch gives security and comfort to the young as well as old. It heals mind and body together. The benefits of massage or touch therapy are well documented in ancient medical texts of China, India, Egypt, Persia and Japan. The earliest surviving text mentioning massage as medicine is the Chinese *Nei Ching* written 3000 years ago.

Ayurveda text from around 1800 BC mentions self-massage with oil as a way of releasing the physical energy. Hippocrates, father of modern medicine, was so convinced with the healthy effects of massage that he wanted all doctors to be trained in this skill. Galen, a famous Roman physician (1st century AD), has written 16 books on massage and exercise.

After a phase of neglect, massage therapy returned to Europe in the 19th century in the form of Swedish massage. In 1994 and 1995 two research studies at Middlesex Hospital and Royal Marsden Hospital in England reestablished the therapeutic value of massage as a relaxing, stress-buster and pain reliever.

Fiona Harrold, the popular author of *Massage Manual,* has scientifically described how massage boosts blood circulation, balances blood pressure, helps digestion, soothes muscles, stimulates the lymphatic system, speeds up disposal of toxins from the body, generates a feeling of well being and triggers the release of endorphins—the pain relieving hormones in the body. It is considered very effective in stress-related problems such as insomnia, headache, high blood pressure, depression and anxiety. It is also used to banish constipation, boost the immune system and relieve pain in sciatica and arthritis. Massage is also *a highly popular, passive exercise.*

Practitioners use a variety of techniques. However, the type most suitable for a person depends on the nature of the problem. Broadly there are five basic modes of massage. These are:

(i) Stroking

(ii) Rubbing;

(iii) Kneading;

(iv) Percussion or tapping,

(v) Vibrating or shaking.

Stroking increases blood circulation, soothes the nerves and is helpful in atrophied skin condition.

Rubbing or friction warms up and relaxes the joints, tendons and muscles, reduces swelling and inflammation.

Percussion relieves muscle atrophy, increases blood supply and soothes nerves.

Vibration is beneficial in neuritis, neuralgia, glandular problems and bowel disorders.

Kneading invigorates muscles, relieves intestinal congestion, and respiration problems.

Body massage is much beneficial in the morning sun. The duration may vary from 15 to 45 minutes. Mustard oil, cotton seed oil and red oil are used for the body, and butter for cheek and neck. Massage should be avoided in serious inflammatory cases, infectious diseases, umbilical hernia, lung infection and after meals.

COLOURS AS SUPPORT THERAPY

It is an age old therapy which was used in ancient Egypt, India and China. It uses solar rays, lights and colours for treating various ailments. The therapy gained scientific acceptance when the *bactericidal action of solar ultra-violet energy* was first discovered in 1877.

Subsequently, psychologists found out the healing effects of coloured lights on body and mind. Blue light was found to have a calming effect, red light having energizing effect, orange stimulated blood supply, violet helped reduce nervous and emotional disturbances, yellow gave joy and happiness and green was a mild sedative. Solar bath itself is highly beneficial to the body.

Methods

In colour therapy, light is applied on the affected parts of the body through various coloured glasses or transparent coloured papers. Sun-charged water in coloured bottles is also used internally and externally. In case of glasses, sun-light is allowed to pass through, and is directed to the body. Such glasses could be placed conveniently at places from where sunlight could pass through and fall on the body for at least 30 minutes.

For sun-charged water therapy, a coloured bottle filled three-fourths with pure water and corked is *placed in bright sunlight for eight hours*. It can be applied on body or taken as a drink. As supportive treatment, a diet containing natural foods of similar colour should be taken. For instance, beets, tomatoes, water melon for red, lemon, grapes, pumpkin for yellow, carrot, mango, orange, ripe papaya for orange and green vegetables like spinach, chaulai, lettuce, etc., for green may constitute such a diet.

Healing Power of Colours

Green For treatment of liver disorders, cold, fever, malaria, ulcers, eye problems, cancer.

Blue Beneficial in asthma, respiratory disorders, high blood pressure, skin problems, insomnia.

Red Low blood pressure, rheumatic disorders, paralysis, tuberculosis.

Orange Kidney and gall stones, hernia, appendicitis.

Yellow Diabetes, abdominal disorders, constipation, throat infections.

Violet Nervous disorders, arthritis, insomnia.

Colour is also considered key to good nutrition. Fruits and vegetables like blueberry, eggplant, black and red grapes, strawberry, red apples, mango, pumpkin, watermelon, carrots, papaya, green peas, spinach etc., that come in deep, vivid hues contain plenty of diseases fighting chemicals called phytonutrients.

ACUPRESSURE

This is a special form of massage in which fingers or finger-like simple wooden instruments are pressed on certain points of the body to *minimize aches, pains, fatigue, tension, stress* and various others symptoms of disease. Unlike acupuncture, in which sharp needlets are pierced into the points in the skin, *Acupressure is non-invasive, safe and simple.* In fact, it is a very natural form of physiotherapy which follows anatomical guides and motor points, stimulation of which relieves various disabilities.

The motor points in the body are not difficult to identity. However, it is always good to initially obtain a proper and professional guidance.

There are small nerves often embedded in or near muscles attached to bones. These are hooked up to various acupressure sites in the Human nervous system. Stimulating these often helps the healing process. Each acupressure site is a cycle about one centimeter in diameter. Pressure is to be applied exactly on this anatomical part for effective results. The finger or knuckle is to be rotated in a narrow circle over this site while maintaining firm pressure.

The Chinese texts on acupuncture have identified over one thousand points or sites on fourteen meridians (or lines) going up and down the body. Acupressure has reduced these to about 60-70 important motor points. It is not necessary to apply pressure or rotational massage on all these points as they are related to various parts of the body and ailments.

Acupressure therapy is useful in pain related to arthritis, elbow, shoulder, neck, back, wrist, knee, ankle and foot ailments, impotence, headache including migraine, sinus troubles, toothache, menstrual problems, insomnia and anxiety, abdominal, chest, urinary, hypertension and constipatory problems. Acupressure cures more effectively in combination with a natural diet and practices. ■

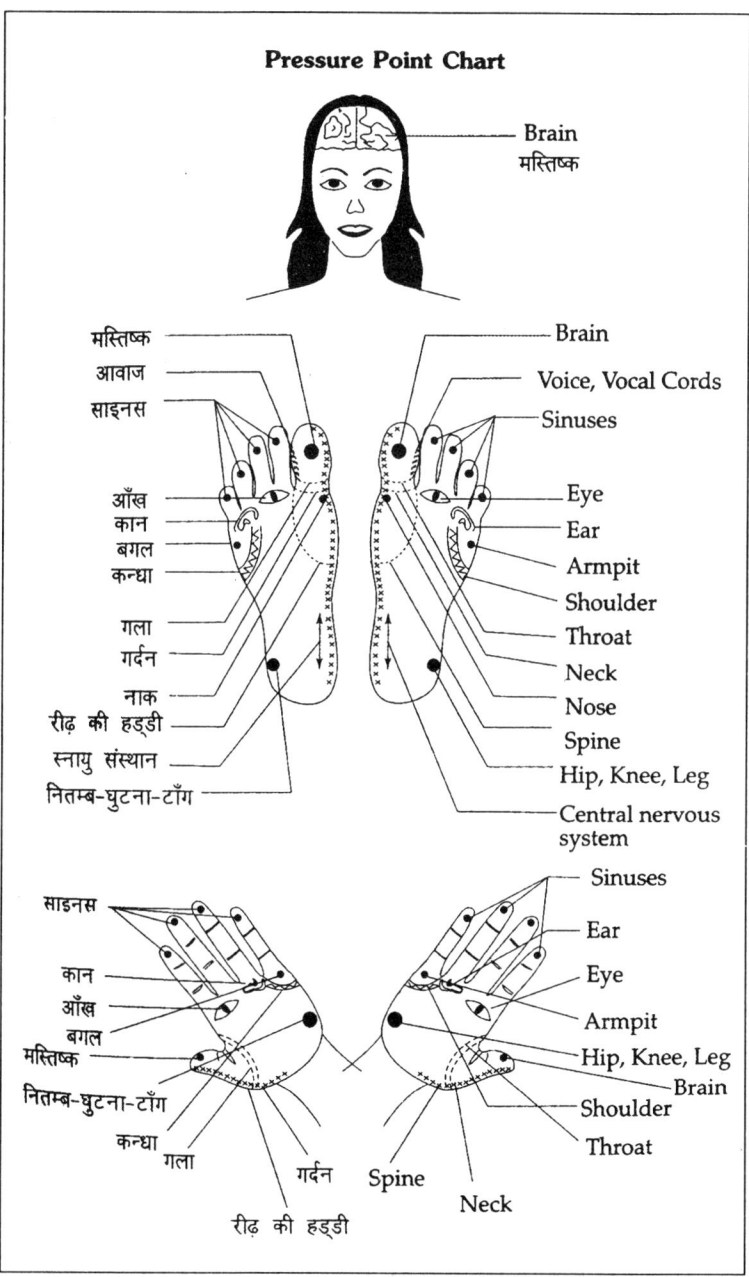

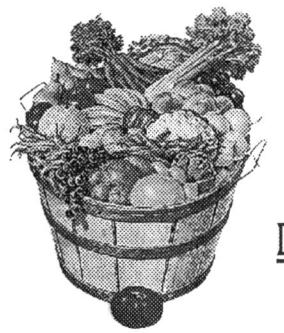

PART 2

FOODS & FITNESS

And God Said: "See, I have given the every herb that yields seed which is on the face of the earth and every tree whose fruit yields seeds to you it shall be for food!"

Genesis 1:29

LIVING FOODS
THE NATURAL MEDICINE

F ood as such has three functions:

(i) It produces energy for work

(ii) It builds body substance and

(iii) Regulates body processes and functions by replacing daily wear and tear of tissues.

In Naturopathy, living food is used as natural medicine against diseases. Food is the first survival need of mankind. "Thy food shall be thy medicine", was pronounced by Hippocraates two millennia ago. Mainstream medical world, of late, has realized the validity of this statement. *Human body is like a temple to which offering of right food should be made in right combination, at right time and with due respect.*

There is a positive relationship between food and health. Human body is build by food, and hence, can be maintained and repaired by food. Fresh natural food with its essential amino acids and enzymes helps body fight against ailments. It is again the food which can restore the acid-alkaline balance in the body that contributes to good health.

Food produced on healthy soil without use of chemical fertilizers, or pesticides is called *nature food*. Many naturopaths call *cutting and cooking as killing the food*. Except Homo sapiens, no other species have a kitchen and they live their full life on raw and ripe uncooked living food in the form of Sprouts roots, fruit, vegetables and cereals. Thus, food which has not been cooked on fire has great value for body. Such foods are nutritionally positive and cannot be over-eaten. In such food, vitamins and enzymes remain intact. There is an English proverb which says : "*God sends foods and Devil sends cooks*".

There are innumerable fruits, roots and vegetables which are eaten either raw or ripe and with full taste. Nature provides such a wide variety of vegetables all year round that one never gets bored of a vegetable diet. Vegetables like tomatoes, cucumber, carrot, radish, cabbage, beet, sweet potato, onion, peas, papaya, lady's finger, pumpkin can be eaten without cooking. *These are pre-cooked by nature on the fire of five elements.* Mint, Coriander, *amla*, tarmarind are consumed raw as chutney. Spinach, *bathua*, *chaulai* (amaranth) and wheat grass juice have great nutritional and curative properties. Peanuts, dry fruit, seeds, dates, raisins are much tastier when taken raw. Green gram, fenugreek (*Methi*), alfalfa and black grams have increased food value when taken in the form of sprouts.

Cooked unpolished rice, whole wheat bread, steamed vegetables, milk and yoghurt can be added to daily diet to *increase palatability. Natural Spices like Haldi (Turmeric), Jeera (Cumin seeds), Dhania (Coriander seeds), Hing (Asafoetida), Adrak (Ginger), Pudina (Mint), Methi (Genugreek seeds), Dalchine (Cinnamon) and coconut milk are not only a pleasure to the palate and nostrils, but have curative medicinal properties.* Where cooking is unavoidable, the loss of nutrients could be minimized by cooking without cutting or cutting in large pieces and cooking at high temperature for minimum time and always using light lid or cover. Steam cooking and using non-stick cookware is a better way of cutting down on fats.

Solar cookers can also be used for natural cooking in which the sun cooks food for us. All fatal ailments yield sooner or later to a natural prescriptive menu than to prescriptive pills.

Frying or deep frying must be avoided. Deep-fried snacks like *bada, pakora, samosa* and *cutlets* not only add lot of fats but pressurize the digestive organs. A safer way is to avoid eating joints, restaurants and eat *home cooked food* as far as possible, consisting of plenty of salads and green vegetables. ∎

HIGH-FIBRE FOODS
NATURE'S SCAVENGERS

THE THREADS or filaments forming the tissue in the plant are called fibre. No plant can stand erect without this fibre. In foods this is the indigestible part popularly known as *roughage*. Neither enzymes nor other digestive secretions can digest it. But, for maintenance of health and prevention of disease fibre plays an important role.

On entering the digestive system, fibre absorbs liquids, mixes with other foods, swells and softens it, gathers these into a mass and winds its way through the intestine and the rectum. It improves the peristaltic movement of the colon, relieves constipation and keeps cholesterol down. It reduces fat intake and all kinds of heart diseases. It aids digestion and fights acute and chronic diseases such as piles, fissure, stomach cancer, varicose veins, etc.

Fibres are two types—*water soluble and water insoluble*. Nuts, legumes, apple, oats, banana and barley, etc., are water soluble, lower cholesterol and control blood sugar levels and diabetes. Soluble fibres are the more civilized cousin of the insoluble fibre as they scrub and *clean more subtly and slowly like a toothbrush*. Water insoluble fibre is found in whole wheat, unpolished rice, grain bran, unprocessed fruit and vegetables like sweet corn, carrot, peas, potatoes. It regulates bowel movement, softens stool and controls constipation. It also protects one from colon and rectal cancer. It dilutes and neutralizes the carcinogens we consume and expels them. The food that is totally devoid of fibre includes meat, fish, egg, fats, sugar and milk products. If one has to take these foods, then they should be adequately supplemented by plant based fibre foods.

Fibre functions as *nature's broom or sponge inside the body* which sweeps and cleans the system of all waste, undigested and morbid matters. Without fibre, food can get trapped in the digestive tract and cause various diseases. While grains alone provide about 35 percent of the fibre in one's diet, fruit and vegetables contribute 47 percent. Together they contribute about 18-20 grams of fibre a day, while the recommended requirement is about 25-30 grams. So, the deficiency could be made up by adding a little more salad or consuming one or two extra fruits.

Because of their high fibre content salads should consist fifty percent of the daily diet. Yet, while eating salads one needs to be very careful. It should be properly cleaned and prepared as some of these may contain a sprinkling of tapeworm eggs and these eggs may grow into larva in the intestine. They burrow through the stomach wall and enter the blood vessel to cause harm to the body. Therefore, salads like carrot and radish should be peeled, cabbage leaf should be cleaned, cucumber properly washed. Avoid eating salads outside.

However, too much fibre may overload the system and make

one feel gassy or bloated. Thus, apart from being judicious in picking the fibre, one should test one's system for about 4-6 weeks to decide the amount that suits one best. It is also important to drink lot of fluids—about 10-12 glasses a day to ensure that the fibre is not trapped in the intestinal tract for want of liquid. Its extra water holding capacity relieves constipation by inducing faster bowel movement. If one wants the inside of the body clean and the outside lean, fibre should be one's first friend in diet.

High Fibre Foods	Percentage of Fibre Content by weight
Apricot (Dried)	24.0
Coconut (Dried)	23.5
Coconut (Green)	13.5
Figs (Dried)	18.5
Figs (Green)	2.5
Dates	7.5
Beans (Baked)	7.3
Beans (Green)	3.3
Barley	6.5
Cabbage (Boiled or Steamed)	8.5
Cauliflower	2.2
Banana	2.0
Almond	14.3
Apple	2.4
Berries	7.3
Corn (Sweet)	5.7

High Fibre Foods	Percentage of Fibre Content by weight
Cucumber	2.2
Carrot	3.0
Lentils	4.4
Oranges	3.0
Onions	2.24
Potato	6.36
Potato (Sweet)	4.32
Rye (Bread)	11.07
Raisins	6.08
Brown Rice	5.5
Spinach (Boiled)	6.3
Tomato	1.4
Wheat (Bran)	44.0
Whole Wheat Flour	9.6
Soyabean Flour	12.0

SPROUTS
THE WONDER FOOD

FROM TIME immemorial sprouts have been advocated as the most nutritious food. Captain Cook sailed in the high seas for ten long years without loosing a single crew member. He attributed the secret of this to a daily ration of sprouted beans. Sprouts are called a wonder food because it contains the largest amount of nutrients per unit of any food known to the mankind till today. It provides all the essential vitamins and minerals and generates powerful and positive chemical changes in the body.

Sprouts produce enzymes, convert starch into glucose, change protein into amino acids, and increase the value of vitamins. According to one study (Dr. Bailey), the vitamin C value of wheat increases 600 times in the early sprouting period. Another report (Dr. Ernest Krebs) states vitamin B increasing 1000 times in the sprouted seed. Wheat sprouts and wheat grass juice are known for their cancer fighting properties. All sprouts are almost predigested and can be easily assimilated by children as well as elderly.

All edible legumes, seeds and grains can be sprouted. Among

these are wheat, moong, bajra, barley, peas, groundnuts, alfalfa seeds, fenugreek seeds, etc. Alfalfa is considered the king of all sprouts. Moong beans, being easily available, are also an excellent sprout food with all vitamins in perfect balance.

How to Sprout

The seeds for sprouts should be washed thoroughly and then soaked overnight in a pot of pure water, properly covered. In the morning, seeds should be rinsed and water drained off. Now the seeds may either be put back in the same pot (up to one-fourth of its size) or tied in a thin and porous piece of cloth to allow the air in. The seeds would germinate and sprout in two days. In winter it may take a longer time. After washing, they may be kept in a refrigerator to retain freshness for days.

H.K. Bakhru (Handbood of Nature Cure) has given an example of how sprouted Moong beans increases the nutrition value:

Protein availability	increases 30 per cent
Calcium content	increases 34 per cent
Potassium content	increase 80 per cent
Sodium content	increases 690 per cent
Iron content	increases 40 per cent
Phosphorus content	increases 56 per cent
Vitamin A content	increases 285 per cent
Vitamin B content	increases 208 per cent
Niacin content	increases 256 per cent

Riboflabin content	increases 515 per cent
Vitamin C content	infinitely

As sprouts absorb a lot of water and contain lot of fibre, it helps in overcoming constipation. Sprouts also reduce gas formation, break down starch into simple sugar, transform protein into amino-acids and fats into simple batty acids.

Sprouts are the real 'Live' food in a combination of fruits and vegetables predigested by nature for human health. ∎

NATURE'S SUPERSTARS

"Leave your drugs in the chemist's pot if you can heal the patient with food."
                                                            Hippocrates

MOTHER NATURE has a series of super foods for protection against health problems. Naturopaths and nutrition specialists have identified the top ones. A selective list is given here:

1. Spinach and Amaranth
   (Palak or Chinese Spinach and Chaulai or Khada)

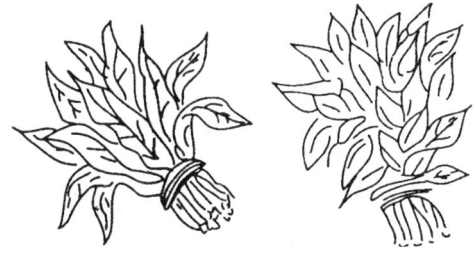

King among the chlorophyll group of vegetables; highly

alkaline. Full of vitamin C and E, protein, folic acid, calcium, betacarotene. Provides protection against cancer, anaemia, acidosis, tooth disorders, urinary and respiratory disorders and stomach ulcers. Considered the broom of the stomach, a friend of the liver.

2. Fig (Anjir)

Highest alkaline effect among all fruits and vegetables. Full of iron, potassium, calcium, chlorine and vitamin A, and digestive enzyme. Its cellulose fibre makes it highly laxative. Effective in asthma, piles and liver disorders.

3. Garlic

Well known for its germicidal and blood purifying qualities.

One normal pod contains more than 15 antioxidants; antibiotic and *bronchial decongestant*. Boosts immunity, lowers blood pressure and cholesterol, reduces blood clotting and prevents cancer. Also prevents hardening of artery that carries blood to the heart. Allicin in garlic works against bacteria, molds, yeast and viruses.

4. Cabbage

Eaten all over the world as a nutritive leafy salad and vegetable, and known for its high mineral, vitamin and alkaline contents. Raw cabbage is excellent remedy for

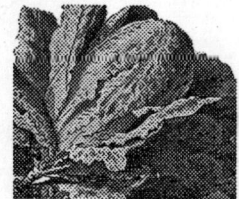

constipation. Its juice is used effectively for stomach ulcers, obesity, skin disorders and premature ageing.

5. Onion

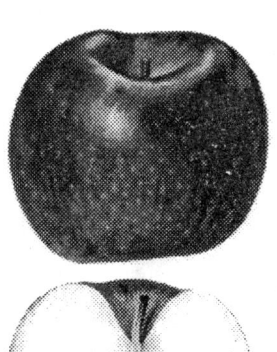

Very important vegetable for nutrition. A good source of potassium, sulphur, phosphorus. Controls high cholesterol, bronchial asthma, sinuses, prevents heart attacks, stomach, rectal and colon cancers. It is a mild acid neutralizer, anti inflammatory, anti spasmodic, carminative, diuretic and aphrodisiac. Remarkable in liver cirrhosis.

6. Apple

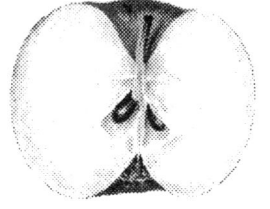

Rich in organic acids. Contains minerals and vitamins in abundance. Highly nutritive and invaluable in maintaining good health. Full of active medicinal properties that help bowel, liver and brain. Full of fibre and low calories. Fights anaemia, dysentery, constipation, heart disease, high blood pressure, rheumatic afflictions, kidney stones, dental disorders and obesity.

7. Stone Apple

(*Bael*)

Its history is traced back to the vedic period. Very rich in fibre, vitamins and mineral contens. Used as sherbet, it has all health giving ingredients. Its leaves also have great medicinal value. Stone apple fights constipation, diarrhea and dysentery, peptic ulcer and respiratory afflictions.

8. Bitter Gourd

(*Karela*)

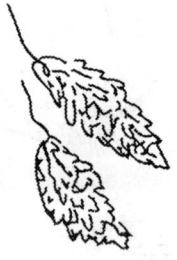

An excellent medicinal vegetable. Contains high dosage of plant insulin. Antidotal, antipyretic, antibilious, laxative and appetizing. It controls piles, blood and respiratory disorders. One of the best missiles in food therapy for diabetes.

9. Whole Wheat and Grass

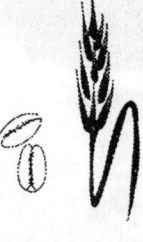

The most common cereal used throughout the world. Contains several medicinal virtues. Every part of it is useful for human body. Helps build and repair muscular tissue. Wheat grass juice is used to fight cancer. Its bran is more useful as roughage and laxative. Rich source of lecithin that keeps body young. Described as a miracle weed, wheatgrass contains a juice having chlorophyll with rich curative properties and adequate amount of vitamins A,B,C,D, and K, alongwith 30 active enzymes. It is also the best anti-oxidant in nature.

10. Beans and Grams

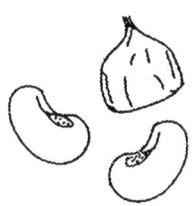
A very good source of B group vitamins. Food value increases amazingly when germinated or sprouted. May lower cholesterol and risk of cancer.

11. Papaya

Known as medical melon of the tropics, papaya is unrivalled by any other fruit. It is alkaline in effect. Papaya has been named as the 'Most Nutritious Fruit' by the Centre for Science, USA. It has a remarkable antiseptic property. It is easily digested and aids digestion of other foods. Normal size papaya has 59 calories, one gram of fibre, folic acid, potassium, very little fat and nearly a day's worth 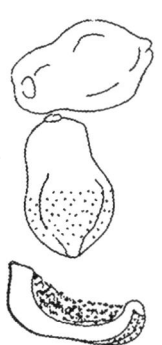 of vitamin C and beta-carotene. Ripe papaya is a laxative, corrects habitual constipation, bleeding piles, chronic diarrhea, menstrual disorders and liver problems. Raw papaya curry and juice correct intestinal disorders.

12. Musk Melon

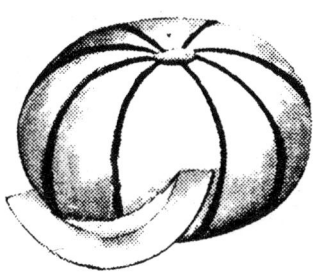
One glass provides 130 per cent of daily value for vitamin C and more than 50 per cent of vitamin A. It provides protection against cancers of the colon and rectum.

13. Bran, Rice

Hundred grams contain more than 20 per cent of the daily value of magnesium and selenium. Its fibre and antioxidant power prevents constipation and colon cancer. Rice bran has 11 times the iron, 45 times the vitamin B-1 and 12 times the selenium content of white rice. Rich source of lecithin, important for body and brain.

14. Tomatoes

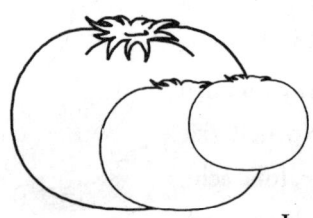

Full of vitamin C (which colours tomatoes red) and fibre, it contains lycopene and helps fight cancer. It is a natural stimulant for kidneys and helps wash away toxins from the body. It adds taste and flavour to all foods.

15. Lemon

Widely sued as a food medicine for its curative properties. Contains pectin and high amount of vitamin C. Helps against cold, circulatory and digestive disorders, obesity, cancer and heart disease. Lemon juice could act as a cheap and affective birth control method and help stop HIV/AIDS growth. Improves immunity. Used as a beauty aid.

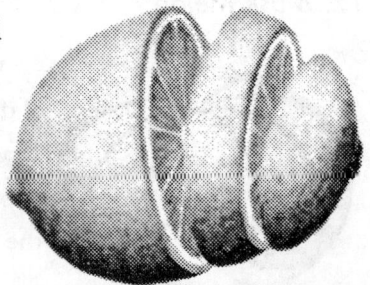

16. Potatoes and Sweet Potatoes

A highly nutritive tuber. Rich in soda, potash, vitamin A and B. Strongly alkaline. Raw potato juice is used as a natural therapy for rheumatism, digestive system disorders, skin blemishes and swellings. Sweet potato (Kandamul) is even more nutritive and used as an excellent food remedy. Rich in vitamin C and E, beta-carotene, fibre, potassium, and iron, it may help prevent cancer.

17. Soya

The Chinese call it yellow jewel. The Japanese consider it the food for both body and soul. It contains phytochemicals, calcium, magnesium, iron and fibre. It may prevent breast cancer and heart disease by decreasing oestrogen levels. Tofu, a curd made from soya milk keeps bones healthy, lowers cholesterol, reduces hot flashes in menopausal women.

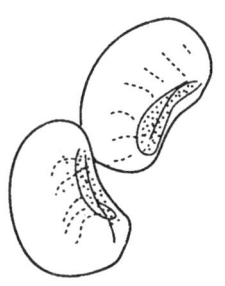

18. Amla

(Indian Gooseberry)

King of vitamin C. Full of minerals and vitamins, its medicinal value is immense. It is laxative and diuretic, fights respiratory and urinary disorders, liver disorders, heart ailments, rheumatism, hair fall and ageing. It reduces body heat and thirst, destroys phlegm and bile and purifies blood.

19. Neem

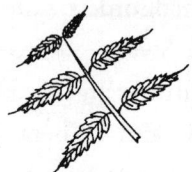

One of the greatest gifts of nature. It fights all fevers and skin disorders, diabetes, asthma, and liver disorders. Neem purifies blood and builds immunity against diseases.

20. Tulsi

(*Holy Basil*)

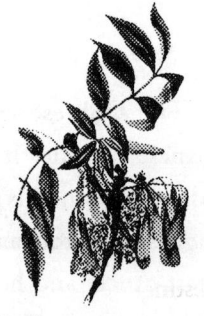

An edible shrub of great medicinal value, unrivalled in religious sacrament and therapeutic applications. It has live mercury in organic form which fortifies the chemical factory within the body. Eliminates bacteria, toxins and poisons, and is effective in controlling cough, cold, respiratory diseases, blood pressure, intermittent and enteric fever, skin, gynaenic and digestive disorders. *Tulsi* improves vision and strengthens the heart. In India, Tulsi is known as the *immortality herb*.

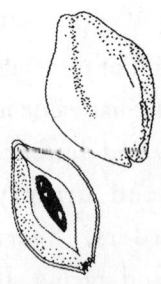

21. Almond

Considered king of nuts, almond is an excellent source of calories and polyunsaturated fatty acids, potassium, magnesium, iron and phosphorus. Three almonds a day (soaked and peeled) enable the body to fight deadly diseases.

Alkaline in effect, it is a great potent tonic. Imparts strength to the brain, increases memory, helps in nervous disorders, insomnia, retards ageing, purifies blood and dissolves phlegm. Almond oil with milk at bed time is a natural laxative.

22. Milk, Yoghurt and Whey

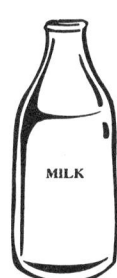

A complete, wholesome food. Contain protein, fat, fibre carbohydrates, all known vitamins, various minerals and all food ingredients required to sustain life. The protein in milk contains all the amino acids essential for body building and repair of body cells (in naturopathic treatment of certain diseases, milk and milk products are prohibited temporarily).

Yoghurt (Curd) is prepared out of milk. It is an excellent health food. It destroys harmful bacteria, protects intestinal tract, improves bowel action, helps in insomnia, hepatitis, jaundice, and promotes longevity. The whey from yoghurt and cottage cheese is also very useful as it contains B vitamins and minerals.

23. Honey

Full of glucose, fructose, sucrose and antioxidants it is nature's sweetest gift to mankind. Contains unique nutritional and curative properties. Prevents cancer and cardiac diseases. Well known for relieving indigestion and headache, it boosts energy, reduces stress, promotes good sleep and relieves discomfort. Honey also disinfects as it contains a germ killer called "Inhibine". The pollen in honey has all the 22 amino acids, 28 minerals, 11 enzymes, 14 fatty acids and 11 carbohydrates.

24. Methi

(*Fenugreek*)

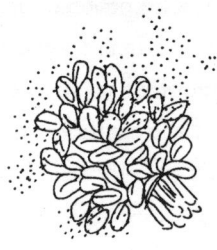

Extremely rich in iron, calcium, sulphur, chlorine, vitamin A and C. Methi leaves are highly alkaline, stops acid build up, stimulates flow of digestive juices, help sluggish liver and lungs and stimulate various organs and nervous system. A natural pain killer.

25. Alfalfa

Contains practically all the vitamins. Contains high percentage of calcium, iron and phosphorus. An Arab saying describes it as a versatile herb, king of all foods and nature's greatest healer. The Herbalist Almanac (1956) states that no other single plant in the vast vegetable kingdom has so many health giving properties. It is the richest land grown source of nutritional trace minerals. It stimulates appetite, helps digestion and improves utilization of food. It build a phenomenal resistance to infection.

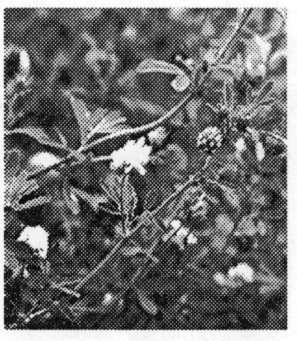

26. Ginseng

The word ginseng means manlike. It is a shrub with a very large root system. Ginseng is a root food and potent tonic that slows ageing, lengthens life, maintains vitality and is used as a special nutritional food supplement. Ginseng tea is recommended for convalescents and old people.

27. Banana

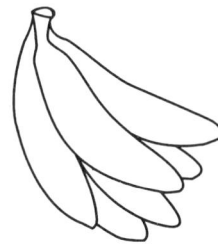

A virtual storehouse of valuable nutrients and nature's best remedy for anemia, diarrhea, as well as constipation. Its inner stem, flower and fruit—raw as well as ripe are full of fibre that binds stool and ease them out. Banana sugar kills microbe and bacteria. Ripe banana with honey is a heart tonic and with milk, a complete food. Banana is rich in solids—potassium, phosphorus, sulphur, calcium, magnesium, iron, copper and iodine. It works wonders for acidity, gastritis, ulcerative colitis, clears intestine. ∎

FACTS ON FATS AND CHOLESTEROL

WITH INCREASING incidence of heart ailments, fats, salt, sugar and cholesterol are under attack. Naturopathy considers salt and sugar, as *white and sweet poison* to be used in moderation, if not avoided.

As eating is also an enjoyable activity, it is impractical to put a complete lid on these items. Some fat is essential in our diet as this is the most concentrated source of food energy (calories). While deciding the amount of fat needed in food, it is necessary to know the basics of calories. *Calories in our foods come from three sources: Carbohydrates, proteins and fats.* One gram of carbohydrate brings in 4 calories and a gram of protein also gives 4 calories. But one gram of fat provides 9 calories.

Our body needs essential fatty acids in small amounts. Fats are mixtures of two kinds of fatty acids:

(i) *Saturated* (butter, coconut oils, red biscuits, chocolates, sauces, puddings, etc.),

(ii) *Unsaturated* (sunflower, safflower, palm oil, soyabean, groundnut oil, nuts, oils fish, etc.).

As fats are loaded with calories, too much leads to overweight and obesity. Saturated fat increases the risk of heart disease and generally a fat-heavy diet also exposes one to the risk of certain types of cancer. So it is wise to cut down on fat and only choose food high in unsaturated fats. In any case, *fat intake should not exceed 15 per cent of one's daily calorific consumption,* or about 40 grams per 2500 calories a day.

Fatty acids in limited quantity are essential to maintain body's oxygen level and are used by the brain, inner ear, adrenal glands and sex organs. The World Health Organization limits daily intake of fats to 300 mg. Dieticians recommend that only 20 per cent of one's total calories should be obtained from fats. In cases like hypercholesterolemia, doctors prescribe not more than 10 per cent.

But the surest way of controlling fat and cholesterol is *sensible eating*. One should eat lots of fruit and vegetables rich in vitamin A, C and E as these are antioxidants. In addition, diets should be full of fibre, as *fibre binds cholesterol* in the intestine and expels it from the body. Cereals like barley and oats, whole wheat flour, brown rice, dalia and wheat bran and green leafy vegetables are full of fibre. So, a vegetarian diet always is the best medicine against high cholesterol.

Dry beans play an important role in protecting the heart and preventing cancer and diabetes. Lentils, black beans, chick peas, moong beans and soyabean lower cholesterol concentration in the body. They contain complex carbohydrates, vegetable protein, dietary fibres, photo chemicals and minerals and, as such play vital role in the prevention of chronic diseases including the one related to the heart. Legumes are not only fat free, but also displace fat from the diet.

Legume-rich diet also works against carcinogenic agents and obesity. One third of all cancers are related to diet.

As cholesterol is abundantly found in meat and animal foodstuffs, non-vegetarians should be discriminating. Red meat should not figure in their diet at all. They should be satisfied with an occasional bit of chicken, or bit of fish as a substitute to meat. Some types of fish contain a type of fatty acid that inhibits formation of blood clots in the arteries.

Cholesterol Content (in 100 grams) of Some Edible Foods	
	(mg)
Egg	550
Crab	125
Mutton	65
Chicken Raw	60
Fish	60
Lamb Raw	70
Liver—Raw	**70**
Pork	**70**
Shrimp	125
Lobster	200
Butter	260
Cream	120
Ice Cream	45
Animal Fats	95
Margarine	65
Whole Milk (Dried)	85
Whole Milk (Fluid)	11
Skimmed Milk Fluid	3
Fruits	**nil**
Vegetables	**nil**
Cereals	**nil**

A *sound dietary habit and moderate exercise* can keep our heart and arteries in good shape and substantially reduce the risk of heart attack. ∎

WHITE AND SWEET POISONS

The word 'salt' came to English from the Latin 'salarium', originally a soldier's salt-money. It was so scarce and prized that part of a Roman soldier's salary was actually paid in salt. In India's freedom struggle Gandhijee's Salt March to Dandi was a land mark symbol of protest against foreign rule.

NATUROPATHS CALL salt and sugar as the two poisons that cause and increase the incidence of diseases. As such, salt is an essential ingredient of life as it flavours and preserves food, maintains blood volume, regulates water balance and nerve impulses. But many people consume salt in excess.

Salt carries 40 per cent sodium and 60 per cent chloride. But only one *teaspoonful of salt per day is adequate* to maintain the level of sodium in the body. Taken in excess, sodium contributes to water retention, high blood pressure, osteoporosis, kidney stones, bronchial asthma, stomach cancer and loss of elasticity in blood vessels, etc. on the other hand deficiency of sodium may lead to nausea, muscular weaknesses, heat exhaustion, mental apathy and respiratory failure. Some studies have shown that use of mineral salt which is a natural product, in place of common salt, reduces the risk of these ailments as it contains beneficial minerals, potassium and magnesium.

One easy way to cut back on sodium is to *change some of the eating habits*. Fresh food contains less sodium than ready-to-cook, processed or preserved foods including potato chips, popcorn, salted nuts, pickles and creams. Almost all fresh vegetables and fruits are *naturally low in sodium* and can fulfil the sodium requirement of the body. These are apple, orange, lemon, grape fruit, berries, pumpkin, beet tops, lentils, cucumber, water melon, lady's finger, almond, walnut etc. It is now a proven fact that industrialized countries which have a higher salt intake in their foods have more hypertension than traditional, low salt primitive societies. There is a popular saying that while ancient Egyptians used oil and salt to mummify the bodies of that dead ancestors, we moderns are now mummifying our living bodies with excessive oil and salt in our foods.

A recent intersalt study of over 10,000 people in 32 countries including India found that the four countries (Indian excluded) with the lowest sodium consumption also had people with the lowest blood pressure. In fact our bodies have not evolved to get rid of excess salt acquired through big salt providing foods like pickles, papads, sauces, chutney, butter, packaged soups, breads, cornflake, samosas, monosodium glutamate.

Like salt, sugar is also detrimental to human health. In obesity, tooth decay, diabetes, acidity, blood pressure, etc. sugar has emerged as the main culprit. Barfi, chocolates, ice cream, biscuits, cakes, pastries, soft drinks, tea and coffee—all contribute to high sugar intake.

While mono-sachharides like fructose (fruit sugar) get digested easily, di-sachharides like white cane sugar need calcium for digestion. Thus affecting teeth and bones. White clarified sugar also increases uric acid in blood leading to gout and high blood pressure. That is why naturopaths prefer molasses (liquid left after white cane sugar has been extracted) which is rich in vitamins B1, B2, and B6.

Like food craving many people have a sugar craving. Researchers say that this craving follows a wave pattern—it escalates to peaks and then subsides. With some determination, it is possible to tone down such cravings for the sake of good health. *Eating sugar is like slow eating of one's own teeth.* One should understand that nature has already provided the needed sugar in grains, pulses, vegetables and fruits and *any sugar we add is extra,* and therefore, not welcome in the body. ■

FLESH FOODS
MYTH AND REALITY

"Good health is primarily the personal responsibility of the individual."

RECENTLY RESEARCH undertaken at the Boston and Stanford universities in the USA has deduced that non-vegetarian food, as against of plant foods and dairy products, is a poor source of minerals, starch or carbohydrates. While animal food and fats have lot of harmful cholesterol and uric acid, plant foods, are generally fat free. Vital fibres are found only in vegetables and some grains. In a recent report brought out by Doctors' Committee on Responsive Medicine, Dr. Neil Bernard, its President has stated with conclusive evidence that beyond whole grains, pulses, green vegetables and fruits human body does not need any additional supplement for complete nutrition—not even dairy products.

Another study covering 3000 men in Finland, Netherlands and Italy showed that lung function (FEV) was found to be the highest in men who ate lots of fruits and vegetables (Reuter).

A recent study published in the American Journal of Clinical Nutrition reveals that the single most reliable way to protect our brain cells and prevent ageing and memory loss is to consume plenty of fruits and vegetables that are full of antioxidants and nutrients.

The word vegetarian or Vegan is derived from the Latin word '*Vegetus*' which means 'whole, sound, fresh or lively'. Nowadays, an increasing number of people are turning to vegetarianism. Most of them are *informed eaters* who have realized that *nutrition is not synonymous with non-vegetarian food and meat is not muscle*. While some think it is cruel to kill and eat animals, others think it is like eating the dead. There are a few who do not approve of *life eating life* and want to draw the line somewhere. But there are also many for whom vegetarianism is more a matter of taste than of conscience or principle. This is reflected in the growing number of 'demivegetarians', who frequently opt for meat free foods but occasionally indulge in meat eating.

Meat eating has a history of its own. Ancient Greeks ate meat with gusto and perceived vegetarians as odd and dangerous. Pythagoras, who turned vegetarian, was ridiculed by hedonistic Romans. While some religions sanctioned meat eating, there were others which propagated a non-violent animistic ethic. In India, during the pre-Vedic period, meat eating was practiced by many. Hunting was a popular pastime among the kings. Yet there were certain sects which practiced strict vegetarianism.

Gandhiji introduced vegetarianism in his ashram as an integral part of his non-violent ethics and practice. Despite spirited advocacy by Milton, Shelley, Newton and Bernard Shaw, vegetarianism failed to win the West for a long time. Now in the

USA and Great Britain the number of people who have adopted vegetarianism in the past decade has exceeded 40 million. More and more people in developed countries are now switching over to green and vegetarian food habits.

One common doubt about vegetarians is that they cannot get enough protein to build muscular strength. Some people probably do not know that one can get more than an adequate amount of protein from a vegetarian diet. Such people should watch more closely the amount of muscle on a 500 lb bull or a similarly massive, muscular vegetarian animal.

In India and many parts of the world, although millions of people avoid meat, vegetarianism became popular only in the latter part of 20th century. Cook books on vegetarian diet are now very popular and supported by medical wisdom, ecology, animal rights advocates, nutrition specialists and naturopaths.

A study of human anatomy and physiology reveals that nature has created the human beings as vegetarian animals as they belong to the herbivorous genus. Endocrinologists say that meat-rich diets dissolve the bones as these are acidic.

Reasons Why Our System is not Built to Eat Meat

Carnivores	Herbivores	Human Beings
Eyes the young ones of meat eating animals can't see for a week after their birth. Developed night vision.	Born with their eyes open and can see immediately.	Born with eyes open. Day vision stronger than night vision.
Teeth Long canine, to seize, hold and tear the flesh.	Front, top and bottom teeth like blades, back teeth like grinders	Teeth like blades and grinders for eating plant food.

Carnivores	Herbivores	Human Beings
Jaws Open wide to capture prey; move up and down, cannot move sideways to grind plants.	meant for cutting and grinding plant food. Cannot open wide enough; can move side to side to grind plants.	Cannot open wide enough but move side to side to grind nuts and vegetables.
Claws Long sharp for attack.	No claws.	No claws.
Tongue Rough, useful for lapping blood, saliva, acidic.	Soft, use lips when thirsty; alkaline, acts on plants.	Soft, useful when thirsty; Saliva alkaline, acts on starches and carbohydrates.
Perspire through tongue.	Perspire through body pores.	Perspire through body pores.
Violent, volatile passionate.	Basically non-violent.	Basically non-violent.
Bowel Smooth, allows food to move along freely.	Full of pouches; meat could get trapped and putrefy.	Full of pouches; meat gets trapped.
Intestines Short; flesh does not remain for very long and meat passes through quickly.	Very long; meat takes time to pass and could putrefy.	Very long; meat could putrefy.
Liver Big livers and kidney; easily throw out waste materials of meat.	Small livers; flesh food puts too much pressure on it.	Small livers; meat puts to much uric acid in blood which gets deposited in joints.
Stomach Highly acidic.	Highly alkaline.	Highly alkaline.
Blood tends to be acidic.	Tends to be alkaline.	Tends to be alkaline.
Instincts Pounce on bleeding prey and kill.	Do not desire to kill small animals.	Feel repulsed on seeing bleeding animals.

It is an established medical fact that feeding on meat regularly produces lots of polyunsaturated fats, cholesterol and calories. These lead to high blood pressure, ulcerative colitis, cancer of the colon and rectum, kidney diseases, arthritis, etc. A recent FAO study has indicated that the growing food scarcity that humanity is likely to face in the 21st century could be solved if people adopt a vegetarian diet. Plants and grains provide twice as much food energy compared to meat, when consumed directly by humans. Meat is known to be an inefficient by-product of food grain as eight kilos of foodgrain produce only one kilo of beef or mutton or flesh food. The quantity of grain required to produce one calorie of beef could produce 10 calories if taken directly.

Many scientists believe vegetables protect against cancer because they contain a wide variety of phytochemicals which are essentially toxins produced to protect the plants. When consumed, these phytochemicals trigger the activity of enzymes that detoxify cancer-promoting compounds in the body. Results of a study released by National Institute of Public Health and Environment in the Netherlands covering 3000 samples in three European countries, i.e. Finland, Netherlands and Italy showed that lung function or forced expiratory volume (FEV) was the highest in people who ate lots of fruits and vegetables. It improved their pulmonary function helping them breathe better and feel better.

However, it should be realized that people develop eating habits during childhood. Various societal and ethnic belief systems also follow food fads and taboos. A true follower of Naturopathy must *avoid value judgment* on eating habits of the people and place the facts before the patient to make an *informed decision*. ■

LEAF LOVERS AND CANCER FIGHTERS

L EAVES CONTAIN almost all the nutrients people need for health. In the tropics like India with plenty of sunshine, rainfall and fertile soil, growing green leafy foliage is very easy. In terms of both dry matter and crude proteins the proportion from green leafy crops is always greater than from any other source.

Research has shown that high intakes of fruits and green leafy vegetables *reduces the risk of all types of cancer.* Leafy vegetables and fruit are potent sources of antioxidants. They protect genetic materials from cancer damage. Fruit and vegetables are also full of thousands of compounds—called phytochemicals. These chemicals stop the growth of cancer cells in the body. Food scientists have identified 14 general classes of anti-cancer photochemicals in fruit and vegetables. These are cruciferous and leafy vegetables like cabbage, amaranth, spinach, cauliflower, broccoli, greens, carrots, tomatoes, pumpkin, melon, cucumber, brinjal, soyabeans and soya products, whole grains, garlic, onions, celery, parsley, citrus fruits, etc.

For instance coriander leaves have a cooling effect on the body and make food digestive. It has high potassium, phosphorus, calcium iron and vitamins A and B. Fenugreek leaves help improve sluggish liver and lungs. Lettuce leaves used as salads are a good source of vitamins A, B, C and E and useful for relaxing the bowels. It is highly beneficial for anemia, acidosis, insomnia, urinary problems and obesity. Spinach is one of the foremost among chlorophyll group of leafy vegetables with molecules similar to the molecule of hemoglobin of our red-blood corpuscles. It is extremely rich in vitamin A and E and its calcium is much readily available than of milk. The organic material of raw spinach leaves is the best for cleansing and regeneration of entire intestinal tract. It is also a protective food for the glands. Amaranth tender leaves like spinach is extremely rich in vitamins and nutrients. It can be used as a staple food, blood cleanser, diuretic, anti-phlegmatic and aphrodisiac. Mustard leaves are the richest known source of dietary lime, high in vitamin A, C, iron and calcium. Tender neem leaves are rich in nutrients and great in cleansing effect and disinfection. Turnip leaves eaten as vegetable have lots of cancer fighting compounds called glucosinolates.

Mint (podina leaves) is known for its curative properties for the last 2000 years. It is full of active enzymes that help in digestive process, regulates menstrual flow, removes abdominal pain and good for hardened arteries and fevers. Indian cuisine is incomplete without curry leaves full of curative properties. Curry leaves (Murraya Koenigi) help ease constipation, asthma, diabetes, digestive disorders, obesity, blood pressure and premature ageing.

A plant-based diet with a variety of such fruit leaves and vegetables, grains and beans, which are naturally low fat and high fibre, reduce the risk of cancer to a great extent and take care of many health problems.

With recent scientific news of *faster post-operative healing among vegetarians,* alternative food habits are steadily catching popular imagination in the West and America. *'Romance with the radish'* and *'Love for the Leaf* are the new buzzwords among the alternative food eaters. ■

CALORIE
THE ENERGY TONIC

A CALORIE IS a unit of heat used to measure the energy value of foods. *Body requires energy to function and the foods provide this energy.* But the calorific requirement is based on age and the nature of work one does. For example, a person doing hard manual labour may require 50 per cent more calories than a person doing a white-collar desk job. Similarly, a person with 40 kg weight is likely to burn two-thirds of calories of a person who weighs 60 kgs (132 lb). The following chart gives an indication of the daily calorie requirement:

Daily Calorie Requirement

Age	Calories Required
Up to 6 months	120
7-12 months	100
1-3 years	1200
4-6 years	1500
7-9 years	1800
10-15 years	2100
16-18 years	2500
Light workers	2200
Medium workers	2800
Heavy workers	3000
Expectant mothers	300 calories *extra*
Lactating mothers	700 calories *extra*

People who become fat and overweight consume more calories than they utilize in their daily work. A basic thumb rule of daily calorie requirement is to multiply one's desirable body weight by 35. Those who do hard physical work or exercise can multiply their desirable body weight by 50 to determine the number of calories required per day.

The accompanying chart gives activity/work-wise calorie expenditure per day.

Calorie Expenditure

Activity	Calorie Expenditure
Sleeping	60
Lying awake	75
Standing	105
Dressing-Undressing	115
Sewing-Tailoring	125
Rapid Typing	135
Light Exercise	165
Walking Slowly	200
Badminton	270
Football	540
Running	570
Brisk Walk	450
Tennis	750
Swimming	500
Hockey	540
Vigorous Exercise	600
Walking Upstairs	1000

Calorie Table of Some Foods

Items	Weight	Calorific Value
Plain Rice	100 gm	175
Curd Rice	100 gm	250
Chapati (5 pieces)	100 gm	350
Cereals and Pulses	100 gm	320
Masala Dosa	one	240
Plain Dosa or Chakule	one	140
Bread	Two slices	150
Idli	One piece	60
Bada Sambar	2 pieces	140
Noodles	100 gm	175
Daal	1 cup	160
Salads	100 gm	35
Apple	100 gm	60
Banana	Large	115
Dates (dried)	4 nos.	100
Figs	2 nos.	100
Grapes	20 nos.	100
Orange/Mosambi	100 gm	45
Mango	100 gm	75
Papaya	100 gm	32
Water Melon	100 gm	11
Green Coconut Water	100 gm	52
Honey+Lemon+Water	200 gm	35
Baked/Boiled Vegetables	100 gm	50-80
Sprouts	100 gm	200
Palak/Chaulai (Spinach)	100 gm	25
Cabbage	100 gm	30
Methi Leaves	100 gm	50
Beet Root	100 gm	43
Carrot	100 gm	48
Potato	100 gm	97
Sweet Potato	100 gm	120
Fresh Green Peas	100 gm	93
Almond/Cashew Nuts	10 pcs	100
Sugar	1 tsp	40
Honey	1 tsp	32
Milk (Cow)	1 cup	130
Milk (Buffalo)	1 cup	210
Yoghurt	1 cup	75
Ghee	1 tsp	50
Butter	1 tsp	35

Ideal Body Weights and Heights

Men		Women	
Height	Weight (kg)	Height	Weight (kg)
5'2"	51–61	4'10'	42–54
5'3"	52–62	4'11"	43–55
5'4"	54–64	5'0"	44–56
5'5"	55–65	5'1"	45–58
5'6"	56–67	5'2"	46–59
5'7"	58–72	5'3"	48–60
5'8"	60–75	5'4"	49–62
5'10"	63–77	5'5"	50–63
5'11"	65–80	5'6"	52–65
6'0"	67–82	5'7"	54–67
6'1"	69–86	5'8"	55–69
6'2"	71–87	5'9"	57–71
6'3"	73–90	5'10"	59–73
		5'11"	61–75
		6'0"	63–78

These tables only indicate the averages. It may be kept in mind that food as such cannot give proper nutrition or energy if taken improperly. It depends on the individual and her/his system as to how much energy it could extract from food and transfer to various parts of the body. Further, persons with different metabolism would burn differing amounts of calories for the same kind of activities.

A recent research at the University of Wisconsin has shown that a life time of restricted calories delays ageing and extends life. A nutritionally balanced and yet calorie reduced diet keeps people younger, more vigorous and less prone to disease. Scientists engaged in finding out new clues about ageing are unanimous about one thing that if you restrict calories, you slow metabolic rate and help organisms live longer. ∎

FOOD FRIENDS

IT IS not enough to eat natural or organically grown foods only. If these foods are not compatible with each other, the process of digestion and assimilation is toned down. About 80 per cent of digestive disorders are caused by eating at a time a variety of incompatible foods. This results in constant battle in the body between different foodstuffs. Complete digestion can be achieved if the food items are similar or mutually balanced. The following tips may be considered:

- Avoid combining protein concentrate with carbohydrate or sugar concentrate foods. This results in indigestion and gas. For instance, eating meat, potatoes, bread, sweets and milk products together would create stomach disorders.

- Protein foods digest better with vegetable salads. Proteins and starches should not be taken at the same meal as digestion of starch is delayed by protein.

- Primary protein foods like seeds, pulses, nuts, soyabean, etc., go well with acid fruits like lemon, sub-acid fruits like grapes, apples, berries, apricots, peaches, etc. Vitamin C in these fruits helps protein digestion.

- Do not mix up protein foods with fat foods in the same meal. They delay the digestion process.

- Avoid mixing carbohydrates and acid fruit in the same meal. It halts conversion of starch molecules into simple sugars. For instance, potatoes or bread do not go well with tomatoes. For the same reason, acid fruits should not be mixed up with sweet fruits; or mango with curd.

- Starches, fats, green vegetables and sugars may be eaten together as all of them require alkaline or neutral medium for their digestion.

- In the same way, protein, green vegetables may be eaten together as all of them require alkaline of neutral medium for their digestion.

- Proteins, carbohydrates and fats should not be taken together. Without protein, carbohydrates take a shorter duration. Fruits take the shortest time. Therefore, it is always good to have a *fruit breakfast, a starch meal with non-starchy vegetables for lunch and a protein meal with non-starchy vegetables and salad for dinner.*

- However, simple meals with smaller number of compatible courses are always better than elaborate meals.

- In this way we can make food our friend and not enemy.

TYPES OF FOODS

Proteins Seeds, nuts, soyabeans, cheese, yoghurt, egg, fish, poultry, meat.

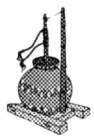
Fats Ghee, butter, oils.

Starch Whole cereals, beans, peas, lentils, potato, etc.

Vegetables

Leafy green vegetables, sprouts, cabbage, cauliflower, green peas, broccoli, tomato, onion, etc.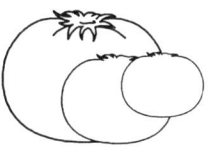

Acid Fruits

Lemon, orange, pineapple, strawberry, berries, grape fruits, etc.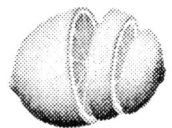

Sub-Acid Fruits

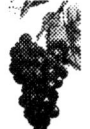 Apples, grapes, mango, guavas, pears, peaches, apricots, plums, raspberries, etc.

Sweet Fruits

Bananas, figs, custard apples, dates, dry fruits, etc.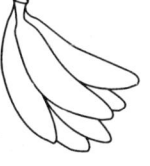

THE SPICES OF LIFE

Although a naturopath always forbids spicy, oily, hot chilly foods, there are a number of spices which are appetizing, digestive, antiseptic and beneficial to health when used moderately and proportionately. *Aniseed (Saunf)* is one such spice. It is cooling and digestive, good for stomach, liver, urinary and menstrual problems.

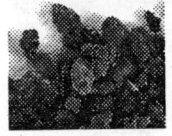

Asafoetida (Hing) is very high in total minerals, calcium and iron. A grain used in food preparations, helps in asthma, bronchitis, indigestion, worms and stomach ailments. *Cumin seeds (Jeera)* is another beneficial spice rich in iron, calcium, potassium, phosphorus, sodium, Vitamin A and B. It is good for diarrhea and dysentery, regularizes menses, improves liver and digestion. *Coriander* (Dhania) widely used in Indian curries is a known food digestive and body coolant in addition to its pleasant aroma and flavour.

Turmeric (Haldi) is often used in vegetables. It heals internal wounds, ruptured muscles and is antiseptic and anticarcinogenic. You can give a powdery end to cuts and wounds by pressing turmeric powder straight into them. *Coconut paste* or milk is used in most parts of south India as a spice for taste and flavour in dishes. It is extremely rich in minerals, full of fibre and laxative. *Fenugreek seeds* are good for digestion and help sluggish liver and lungs. *Black pepper (Kali mirch)* is known for its digestive properties, iron, phosphorus and carotene. *Saffron (Kesar)* is an important and useful spice for rheumatism, loss of appetite, liver, spleen and urinary infection, in addition to its aroma and colouring effect on food. *Cinnamon (Dalchini)* is another natural spice that gives flavour, improves taste, digestion and reduces cold. Like cinnamon, *Cloves (Laung)* also has an aromatic effect. These are good for oral hygiene and toothaches, and are used as food preservatives.

Ginger (Adrak), used both in food and as medicine, is a potent anticoagulant, digestive, anti-flatulent,

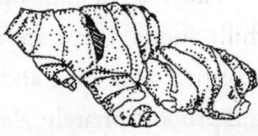

anti-inflammatory, anti-carcinogenic and very good pain killer for osteoarthritis. Ginger boosts circulation by stimulating central nervous system and dilating blood vessels. The uses of *onion and garlic* have already been mentioned in this book. Now research has shown how garlic suppresses human colon cancer cell, reduces LDL-cholesterol and inhibits development of tumour cells, bronchitis and sinusitis.

Mustard seeds reduce muscular pain, worm infections, food poisoning and work as food preservatives and beauty aids.

Mint (Pudina) is another popular, medicinal spice. It is valued as a carminative, antispasmodic, digestive and appetizing. *Poppy seeds (Khaskhas or Posta)* not only increase the taste of food but help in insomnia and sunstroke. *Ajwain* is known for its action in digestion, cold and cough and toothache.

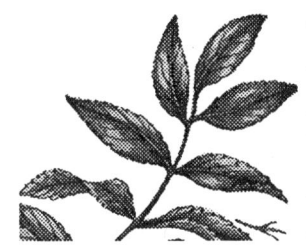

South Asian and East Asian kitchen are full of such spices and herbs used as cooking ingredients, but also having great healing powers.

These spices when used judiciously are health-giving. Apart from titillating the taste buds, many of the spice plants contain very powerful, antibiotic natural chemicals capable of either killing or neutralizing the bacteria and fungi that commonly contaminate the foods.

Even animals are greatly benefited by eating such plants having strong anti-microbial potency. In a way, these are nature's antibiotics against diseases. About 80 per cent of the recipes in tropical and sub-tropical countries are prepared with spices like onion, garlic, ginger, turmeric, black pepper, capsicum, mint, coriander, cinnamon, cloves, saffron, cumin seed, fenugreek and aniseed. If selectively used, these are *in fact the spices of life*. ■

NATURE DIET FROM NATURE FARM

NOWADAYS IT is extremely difficult to get naturally and organically grown food. Mother nature has been greatly harmed by human knowledge, action and intervention. The misguided methods of crop and vegetable cultivation, use of chemical fertilizers, pesticides, herbicides, hormones and soil conditioners continue to destroy our land and vegetation. As a result, people are forced to eat unnatural and synthetic food products which lead to pesticide and agro-chemical residue in their blood. This is nothing but slow poisoning of the body. Even synthetic milk is now sold in the market further adding to this poisoning.

The healthiest food is that which is grown without chemical fertilizer, pesticides, herbicides and hormones. Such food crops are allowed to grow naturally as trees in the forest and mountains. A gram of natural soil contains about 100 million nitrogen fixing bacteria and other soil enriching microbes. So there is no need to damage and destroy the physical texture and micro nutrients of the soil with fertilizers and chemicals. Also by pounding and kneading the soil repeatedly like bread dough, we drive out the humus and air so essential to micro organisms and in this process render the soil barren and devoid of life. Then we try to plant trees in this lifeless soil and add chemical fertilizer forcing these to grow as we wish.

Masanobu fukuoka, the famous green philosopher and practitioner of nature farming in his book, *The One Straw Revolution,* has suggested four basic principles of nature farming. These are:

No Cultivation: No ploughing or repeated turning of the soil and instead allowing the millions of microbes and earth worms to do the job of tilling.

No Chemical Fertilizer: The straw and leaves after harvest should be allowed to decompose in the field itself as green manure. A little poultry or cow dung added to it can get high yield.

No Deweeding: Weeds decrease when cultivation is discontinued. If seeds are sown while the preceding crop is still ripening in the field, those seeds would germinate ahead of the weeds.

No Pesticides: Spraying pesticides creates conditions for more pest attack. The best away is to promote biological control of pests.

The growing of vegetables, grains and fruits by this method is the best way to obtain natural food. However, it may not be possible for everybody to practice nature farming. In order to minimize the intake of unnatural food, some vegetables like gourd, bitter gourd, cucumber, papaya string beans, *palak,* etc., can be grown in the backyard or terraces.

While animals are born with an instinctive ability to distinguish between what they should or should not eat, this instinct does not go beyond man's infancy. Then women and men start *feeding with their head rather than mouth* according to their impulse, taste, fancy, flavour and hunger hormones in the brain.

Instead of producing natural food, emphasis is now on the food processing industry. Our shelves are now overflowing with bottled foods, canned foods, frozen and dried foods, instant soups, breakfasts and dinners packed in polythene bags. Food today is not considered as a critical source of life support, but something that pleases the palate and titillates the senses. Followers of Naturopathy should always look out for nature food, promote nature farming and prevent erosion of natural soil.

It may be remembered that nature diet or food does not mean only organically grown food. Being part of nature we should adjust our diet to the natural cycle and seasons instead of our diet drawing us away from nature. Food is not only physiological, it also influences our emotional and spiritual life.

Fukuoka divides food into four main classifications:

1. A lax diet conforming to habitual desires and taste preferences, called self-indulgent, empty eating.

2. The standard nutritional diet based on biological conclusions or could be called materialistic, scientific eating.

3. Diet based on spiritual principles and idealistic philosophy called diet of principle.

4. The read natural diet following the will of heaven or nature discarding all human knowledge. This food unites body, mind

and heart. "People do not create food from nature; heaven bestows them." And therefore, the body should be helped and allowed to choose its own food from nature that suits it the best.

The "SAMBHAV" nature farm in Orissa (Rohibanka) and the Gloria Nature Farm near Pondicherry have been doing pioneering work in promoting these ideas. More and more organizations are joining this movement to protect the common property sources of nature and the mother earth which provide us nature food. ∎

FITNESS FOR FREEDOM

LIFE IS work, motion, movement and mobility. In fact, our bodies are made by nature for regular movement and vigorous exercise. Fifty per cent of the body is made up of muscles. Exercise makes these stronger.

- But we should not confuse exercise wit activity—although both are importan Activities use the body for a specifi purpose, i.e., to work for a living. On th other and, exercise is meant to maintai the body and keep it fit for working an living.

- So it is a long term investment to kee the body free from diseases and make self-dependent. With physical fitnes through exercise, one can lead a life of *real freedom in old age without seeking help and support from others for doing ordinary everyday help and support from others for doing ordinary everyday tasks.*

- Regular exercise has proven benefits in prolonging life, preserving the suppleness and flexibility of the body and strengthening the joints. It is said that one is as young or as old as one's joints. Exercise keeps one active and fit.

- Exercise not only makes one feel good but also makes one look good. It improves one's overall personality. Body becomes lighter, steps stronger, mind becomes alert, endurance grows, tension reduces, ability to cope with stress increases, one feels more youthful, and enjoys life better. Working out also works wonders in bedroom giving a great boost to the libido and life itself.

- There is a *positive connection between exercise and a healthy heart.* Studies have shown that a less active person has *three times higher risk of heart attack* than an active and hardworking person.

- A physically fit person is also less likely to develop hypertension. Exercise also makes kidneys, lungs and bowels efficient, improves blood circulation, prevents lung congestion, intra-intestinal gas formation, constipation and vitalizes the respiratory system.

- Sweating in exercise helps the kidneys to eliminate waste matter from the body. It also improves the taste for food, helps digestion, promotes physical strength and mental vigour. *It makes one eat less and weigh less.* Studies suggest that people who are moderately active eat less than people who are sedentary.

- Exercise is also *nature's remedy against depression and stress.* Those who have a history of heart disease, high blood pressure, dizzy spells, blackouts, persistent back trouble and are convalescing, need to consult a doctor or fitness expert about the correct exercise schedule.

Fitness for Freedom

- The easiest, the best and the most enjoyable form of exercise is *walking briskly in the morning for about 40 minutes.* Pre or post dinner walks are also useful.

- Jogging is another exercise that give *more points in less time.* Running on flat surface is still better. *Cycling* outdoors is very good for bones and joints.

- *Swimming* is next in importance after walking as it involves the whole body. *Skipping* is also an excellent aerobic exercise beneficial for cardio-vascular fitness. *Aerobic dance,* evolved recently, makes fitness enjoyable.

- Then there are *strength and stress exercise* that keep our necks, backs and joints in good shape. Even short bouts of 15 minutes each for cleaning the house, gardening and playing with kids has a heart-healthy, mood-boosting effect on body and mind.

- In all exercises, one should *keep two things in mind:*

(i) The location should have enough fresh air and greenery, and

(ii) An exercise should enable one to perspire.

- In Indian mythology, Hanuman is admired as a great athlete. In ancient China, Priests used to prescribe 'Cong Fou', a series of ritualistic exercises for relief of pain and ailments. Ancient Greeks had their God of Health (Aesculapius) and were keeping their bodies fit, flexible and beautiful.

- Yoga in India was developed to unite body and mind for freedom from worldly pain. ■

EATING PLAN AND DETOX DIET

WE EAT to nourish our body, preserve our health, satisfy hunger and yet eating disorders have emerged as a major threat to human health. In fact, *how, what and when one eats decides the health status of a person.* Naturopaths, dieticians and nutrition specialists all agree on the need for an individual eating plan. They suggest that such a plan should divide the day into morning, afternoon and evening. *During this period one should have three servings of legumes or grains, two servings of fruit and dark green leafy vegetables, and one serving of low fat dairy products like milk, buttermilk, yoghurt.*

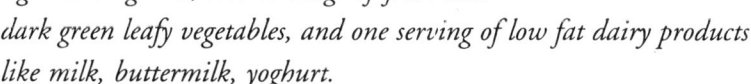

The diet of active women and men interested in losing weight should not consist of more than 1200 calories a day that contain a balance of carbohydrates, protein and essential fatty acids. Fruit with high vitamin C content has fat fighting properties. It has been calculated that if one cuts out three rounded teaspoons of sugar from daily tea, it saves 96 calories a day or 35,000 calories per year.

Cutting down calories requires a judicious eating habit. However, *it is advisable to eat the bulk of the calories during the day and before the sunset.* Avoid eating out and if the lifestyle dictates eating out, be extremely judicious in selecting foods low in fat and high in fibre, vitamins and minerals. Junk food at eating joints like *chaats, chips* and *pakoras* are, in fact, dead foods that harm the health of a person.

Food can be enjoyable and nutritious if properly and carefully prepared. It adds to our happiness and satisfaction. One of Japan's eating aphorisms for instance, says "Happy eating makes for happy family life…., treasure family taste and home cooking". It advises people against eating out where you have no control over the quality of food you eat.

There is an English proverb which says: "The glutton digs his grave with his teeth." Many people do not experience hunger as they tend to eat quite often. Colleen Pierre, a Baltimore dietician uses an acronym, HALT, to help people focus on why they are eating. In HALT, H stands for hunger. So if you are really hungry, go ahead and Halt if you are Angry, Lonely or Tired. Proper chewing of food is also very essential. In fact one should chew food as many times as the number of teeth one has. Since eating is useless without hunger and digestion, it is more important how you eat than what you eat. Respect your digestive tract more than the food. Give it time to gear up and set to work. It also needs rest after the work. Thorough chewing helps in this process. It breaks down solid food particles, produces saliva enzymes, the first digestive juice for food and keeps the teeth sharp, clean and active. Indigestion, heartburn and acidity are caused by inadequate chewing of food.

The natural principle of eating is: *'Drink your solid foods and eat your liquids'.*

While eating one must also sit properly so that the stomach has the space it needs to function and facilitate the digestive process. Leave the dining table when you are three quarters full. To kick start appetite and the digestive process a piece of ginger with a pinch of salt should be taken 10 minutes before the meal. The most natural way of stimulating digestion is to avoid overeating.

It takes about two to thirty five hours for food to pass through and clear out of one's system depending its type, quantity, fibre content and water you drink during the day. The lighter the food, the quicker it gets out of your system with help of fibre and water.

Once a while the body also needs to be cleansed of accumulated toxins caused by dietary indiscipline and life-style blues.

Breathing polluted air, exposure to radiations, partying, intake of caffeinated and processed foods, alcohol, non-veg food, excess fat, salt and sugar produce toxins in the body leading to fatigue, lethargy, low vitality and energy. As most of the toxins are housed in fatty tissues a rise in the toxin level also leads to a simultaneous rise in body weight. Therefore, the system needs to be detoxified and revitalized.

Consult a naturopath for appropriate detox diet to get rid of the toxins from our body. Do not take to frequent enemas or fasting as these might cause loss of essential nutrients. Usually a detox breakfast should consist of a glass of lemon water and 2 or 3 fruits. The lunch should consist of partly steam boiled vegetables preceded by raw salads, followed by some dry fruits like dates and finished with a glass of vegetable juice (beetroot, carrot, tomato, spinach, khira, pineapple, etc.). Dinner may consist of salads, a jowar or bajra chapatti and steamed vegetables. Between these meals drink plenty of liquids, boiled water, coconut water, lemon water, distilled butter milk. Exercise long brisk walks, sauna, massage and steam bath supplement the detox process further. The process always starts with an enema and continues up to 5 to 7 days. Return to normal diet gradually over the next five days. ■

YOGA
HEALING MIND AND BODY

THE NATURAL healing powers of yoga are now universally accepted. Scientific research on yoga around the world has proved its efficacy as the *best form of exercise that unites mind and body and keeps muscles, joints and other organs of the body in fitness.*

There is a developing branch of psychology popularly known as *bioenergetics* which recognizes the close relationship between body and mind. It has proved how the body's respiration and metabolism create energy for physical movement and influence thoughts and emotions. However, the ultimate aim of yoga is to transcend body and mind and live in complete spiritual harmony with the self and soul.

There are four yogic paths known as:

(i) *Karma Yoga* (Selfless action and service);

(ii) *Bhakti Yoga* (Devotion with humility);

(iii) *Raja Yoga* (Physical and mental control), and

(iv) *Janana Yoga* (Study, reflection, meditation).

Yoga also has eight limbs (Astanga) known as:

(i) *Yama* (Social and ethical discipline);

(ii) *Niyama* (Personal discipline);

(iii) *Asana* (Body postures);

(iv) *Pranayama* (Control of breathing);

(v) *Pratyahara* (Mind control);

(vi) *Dharana* (Concentration);

(vii) *Dhyana* (Meditation), and

(viii) *Samadhi* (Super-conscious state).

Of these, the most popular and widely known parts of yoga comprise the yogic *kriyas, asanas and pranayama*. They energize the body and mind, improve blood circulation, digestion, respiration and excretion and promote inner health and harmony. They also slow down the process of ageing.

Yogic exercises should be performed in a clean, quiet and well ventilated place with fresh air. Morning or evening, when the stomach is empty, is the best period. The duration may be between 30-40 minutes. The exercises should be performed on a clean mat or blanket (during winter) covered with a cotton sheet. Clothing should be loose and light. The diet should be plain and bland with plenty of vegetables, fruit and salads. During pregnancy *asanas* should be avoided. Persons suffering from blood pressure, heart troubles or serious organic diseases should consult a doctor or a yoga expert before starting *asanas*.

KRIYAS

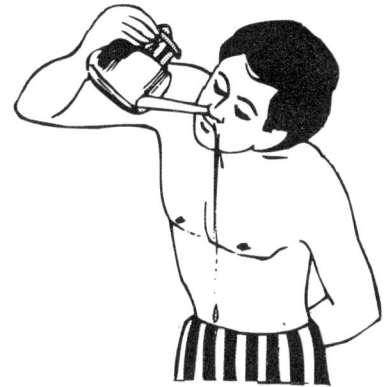

Kriyas, an integral part of yoga, have great therapeutic value. These are very effective in cleansing the body. There are six such cleansing techniques of which two, namely, *Jalneti* and *Kunjal* or *Voman Dhouti* can be practiced very easily and safely.

Jalneti cleanses impurities of nose and throat, cleans the air passage of the nostrils with tepid saline water. Nowadays *Jalneti* pots are available in market or at nature cure and yoga centres. Take such a pot, put half a teaspoonful of salt and fill it with clean, lukewarm water. Insert the nozzle of the pot into the left nostril, bend the head backwards slightly, and allow water to flow out of the other nostril slowly. The process can be reversed. During this process inhaling or exhaling should be done through the mouth only. *Jalneti* should be practiced in the morning. This *kriya* improves the vision, cools the head, relieves headache, cough and cold, sinusitis, migraine and other inflammations. In the beginning, *Jalneti* should be done under an expert's guidance.

The other popular *kriya* known as *kunjal* is to cleanse the stomach. Early morning after going to toilet, drink four to six glasses of lukewarm water with a little salt mixed in. Stand erect, bend forward and insert middle and index fingers (of the right hand) into the mouth until they touch the uvula. Tickle it until there is a vomiting sensation and the saline water comes out. The process of tickling (the uvula) should continue until all the water comes out. This *kriya*, done once a week, improves digestion, cleanses the stomach of excessive bile, reduces constipation and gastric problems. No food should be taken immediately after this *kriya*. People with high stomach ulcer, heart or hernia problem should avoid this *kriya*.

ASANAS

In addition to *kriyas, asanas* (body postures) are very important in maintaining good health and immunity against disease. They work mainly on the endocrine and nervous systems. There are about 64 varieties of *asanas* out of which the following are briefly mentioned here. It is always wise to start with the simpler ones and then take up the others. Initially, guidance of a yoga expert is necessary as wrong practices may be harmful.

Padmasana (Lotus Pose)

Sit straight with legs stretched. Bend the left leg and place it on the right thigh. Similarly, place the right leg on the left thigh. Place the palms on the upturned heels below the navel. Duration 1-2 minutes.

Benefits: This posture is very good for meditation and *pranayam*. It helps in the treatment of spine, heart, lung and digestive disorders.

Halasana (Plough Pose)

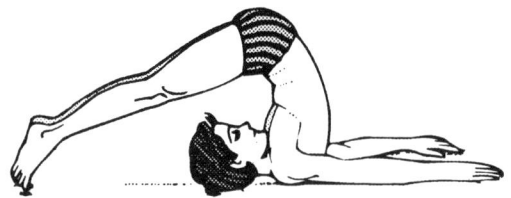

Lie on the back with feet together. Keep the palms alongside the thighs. Inhale and raise the right leg without bending knees. Exhale and bring the leg down. Follow the same process for left leg also. Then raise both the legs slowly and gradually to angles of 30 degrees, 60 degrees and 90 degrees. Bend them over head without bending knees. Move them further until they touch the ground. Hold on to this posture for 15 seconds to 3 minutes, breathing normally.

Benefits: Relieves tension in the back, neck and legs. Beneficial in the treatment of lumbago, spinal rigidity, rheumatism, arthritis, sciatica and asthma. An excellent exercise for the pelvic region. Burns excess fat on the thighs, hips and abdomen.

Bhujangasana (Serpent Pose)

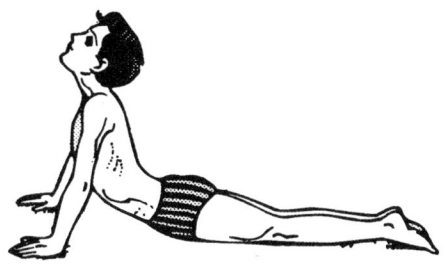

Lie on stomach with legs straight and together and toes pointing backwards. Place palms below the shoulders and arms by the side of the chest. Inhale and slowly raise the head and upper body (head, neck and chest). Look up as far back as possible for a few seconds. Exhale and come back to original position. Repeat 3 times.

Benefits: For cervical spondilitis, bronchitis, asthma, eosinophilia; good for back muscles, vertebra, abdomen and the reproductive system.

Dhanurasana (Bow Pose)

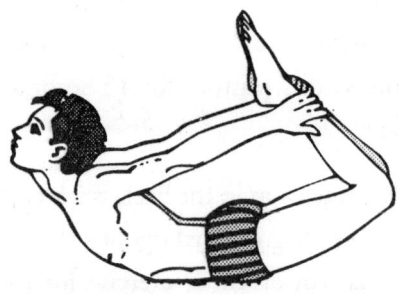

Lie down on stomach. Bend legs towards the hip. Hold them firmly by the hands. Inhale and raise the thighs, chest and head for 10 seconds. Repeat twice.

Benefits: Abdomen, navel and chest muscles become strong. Spine becomes healthy and flexible. Good for relieving flatulence, constipation and menstrual irregularities. Prevents sterility.

Pachimottamasana (Posterior Stretching Posture)

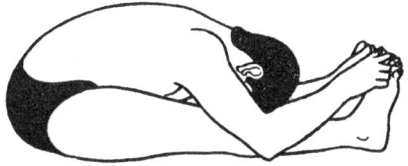

Sit erect with legs stretched forward and close. Bend forward slowly with hands stretching forward. Make the face rest on or bend over the knees and palms holding/touching the feet. Come back to original position after a few seconds. Repeat twice.

Benefits: Fine stretching exercise. Improves abdominal functions and respiratory system.

Vajrasana (Pelvic Pose)

Sit on legs bent backwards. Keep the knees together. Let both the hips rest in between the heels. Place hands on thighs. Keep trunk and neck erect.

Benefits: This *asana* is most beneficial after meals. It improves the digestive capacity.

Chakrasana (Wheel Pose)

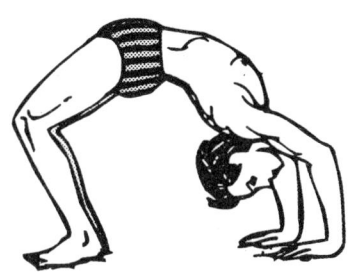

Lie on the back. Raise the whole body upwards resting on feet and palms curving the spine. Stay for a few seconds and slowly come back.

Benefits: Strengthens vertebral column, increases oxygen intake capacity. Prevents respiratory disorders. Relieves stiffness of joints, back, shoulder, thoracic cage and helps in the treatment of asthma, constipation and obesity.

Ardha Matsyendrasana (Spine Twist Pose)

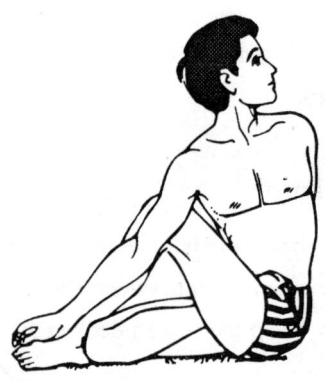

Sit erect stretching forward the legs. Bend the right leg and place the heel under the left hip. Similarly, bend the left leg, cross it over and place the foot beside the right knee. Try to hold the left ankle by passing the right arm over the left side of the left knee. Stay in this posture for a while. Repeat the same process on the other side.

Benefits: Ensures free movement of spine—massage liver, spleen, bladder, pancreas, intestine and other abdominal organs.

Helps in the treatment of obesity, dyspepsia, diabetes and urinary disorders.

Sarvangasana (Shoulder Stand)

Lie flat on back with arms by the side. Bring legs up slowly to 90 degrees angle and them raise the rest of the body by pushing the legs up and supporting the weight of the body with hands. Body may be kept as vertical as possible. Stay in this position for 2-3 minutes. Come back to original position slowly.

Benefits: This exercises the whole body, improves blood circulation, relieves bronchitis, dyspepsia, varicose veins and improves digestion. Stimulates thyroid glands and influences brain, heart and lungs. Not advisable in high blood pressure.

Shavasana (Relaxed Pose)

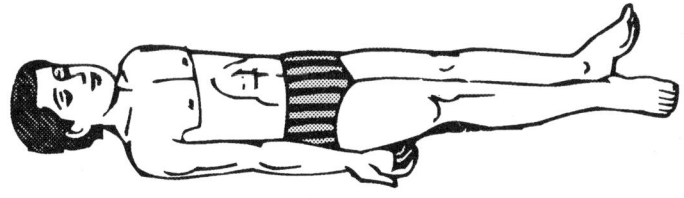

Lie flat on the back comfortably. Loosen all parts of body to achieve complete relaxation. Keep mind free from all thoughts. Concentrate on rhythmic breathing. Remain motionless in this position for 10 minutes. This *asana* is done at the beginning and end of all *asanas*.

Benefits: Highly beneficial to people busy in mental activity like reading, writing etc. Reduces high blood pressures, eases tension, stress and physical exhaustion, soothes nervous system.

All these *Asanas*, if practiced regularly, would not take more than 30 minutes a day and have the power to protect the body from many diseases.

Pranayama

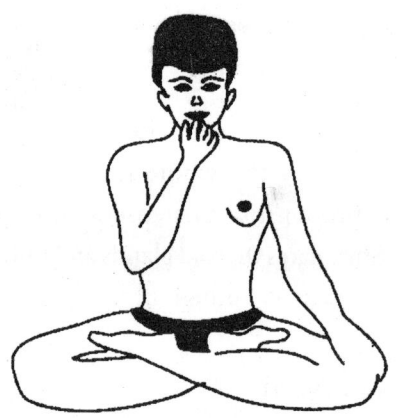

In yoga '*Ayma*' means control or regulation. Thus, *pranayama* means regulated breathing. The process of *pranayam* involves controlled inhaling and exhaling or rhythmic breathing. It activates respiration and strengthens heart and lungs. Deep breathing of fresh air during a brisk morning walk gives new life to the body. There are various types of *pranayama* known as *Anuloma-viloma, Bhastrika, Sheetali, Sitkari, Suryabhedan, Bhramari,* etc.

The most common, simple and easy method is *anulomaviloma* or *nadisudhi pranayama*. For this sit in *padmasana* or any comfortable meditative pose keeping head, neck and spine straight.

Place the left hand on the left knee. Close the right nostril with right thumb. Breathe out slowly through the left nostril. Now, inhale slowly and deeply through the left nostril, keeping the right nostril closed. Then close the left nostril with the little finger and ring finger of the right hand and exhale through the right nostril. Then inhale through the right nostril keeping the left nostril closed and exhale through the left. Repeating this cycle ten times would purify the heart and lungs and calm the nerves.

It helps in controlling asthma, improves working of liver, pancreas and kidney, and stimulates the system. The ratio of inhaling and exhaling should be 1:2. This means exhaling should always take double the time taken for inhaling. In popular idiom, the process is called *Puraka* (inhalation) *Kumbhaka* (retention) and *Rechaka* (exhalation). While *puraka* enlarges the chest cavity and fills the lungs with fresh air, *kumbhaka* increases the carbon dioxide level in the blood, promotes absorption of oxygen and toning of tissues. *Rechaka* forces out toxins and impurities from the body. As it improves concentration of mind, spiritual people do mediation with the help of *pranayama*.

MEDITATION

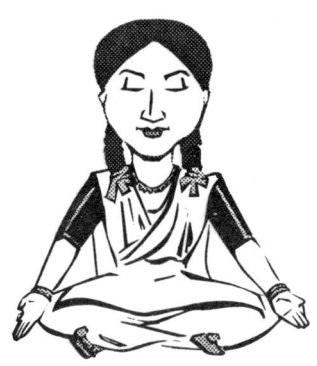

A journey of the self through self, meditation is the next step to *pranayama* to recontact your source of awareness in silence. As life becomes complex, tense and stressful, the natural balance between body, mind and spirit decline. Meditation is the medicine that restores this balance through a journey into the true self. There are various methods of meditation. Some begin with the heart, others with head, some move up through the six chakras—starting with Muladhar and ending with Sahasrar in the head. Yet most of the experts recommend watching one's own respiration as the starting point and then go through a journey of self-discovery from the known to the unknown. Respiration is a unique tool for leading the journey, as it can be either conscious or unconscious. So none can start with the conscious and from there, advance toward the subtler truth about oneself and finally realize the unity of self with the divine. In his Yoga sutra, Sage Patanjali says: By observing and listening to the breathing, we can observe our thought process in the mind. Those who do not believe in the divinity can discover through meditation the phenomenon of mind and matter – the innumerable biochemical and electromagnetic reactions constantly occurring through out, inside the body and their relationships with the known self.

All meditations begin with a prayer for peace of mind and peace in the world. Open your heart to God and invite him to come and reside in it. Hold His hand and go beyond the world, beyond the self, beyond thought. Remain with Him as long as you could – effortlessly. ■

POSITIVE THINKING

IT HAS been discussed at the beginning, how human health is a condition of physical, spiritual and social well-being. *Health leads to happiness as much as happiness leads to health.* When we are happy, we think better, feel better and work better.

Real happiness comes out of pleasant and positive thoughts and certainly not from criticism, blaming, accusing or attacking. And positive thoughts always emanate from rational thinking. If we cultivate the habit of thinking positively we can overcome frustrations, despair and despondency. If we decide to be negative, rude, irritable, impolite, aggressive and harmful, these would destroy us, our health, family and the society around us.

All the remedies in Naturopathy would fail to cure the disease of negative thinking, pessimism, suspicion and self-pity and delusions of persecution. Most of the diseases around the world are psychosomatic. For curing the mind one should be one's own doctor. We should always keep in mind that the greatest success in life is simply being happy. If we think happy thoughts we become happy, and if we think positively, we become positive. Positive thinking begins the day we stop crying wolf or finding fault with others and start discovering goodness in the others. Negative thoughts aggravate our stress level, overload our system and lower our immunity and ability to fight the diseases. On the other hand, positive thinking always boosts the body's defenses and immunity. Positive thinking also promotes strength in an individual.

Positive thinking has a positive impact on our health. Our nervous system receives thousands of negative stimuli from outside. Positive minded people resist these stimuli with positive thoughts and actions:

- If the glass is half empty, they see it as half full.
- They are not cynical or suspicious.
- They develop a positive mental attitude through positive perception and self-image.
- They keep the windows of their minds open on all matters and do not jump to conclusions.
- They stand up for their convictions and do not compromise for convenience.
- They accept and create challenges at home, workplace and in social life.
- They are not afraid of taking full responsibility for their thoughts and deeds.
- Positive people have greater biological efficiency, less disease, better sleep and increased emotional intelligence.
- They are not swayed by emotions and excitement.
- They do not appropriate the achievements of others as their own, and instead, appreciate others' contributions.

- They encourage, motivate and recognize the worth of others at every opportunity.
- They are not envious of their colleagues and friends.
- They always want to do more and do better.
- They like innovative approaches to traditional problems.
- They dislike to be part of a problem and prefer being a part of the solution.
- They prefer to show by example and actions rather than words.
- They feel happy seeing others fulfilling themselves.
- They respect difference, accept change and encourage communication, conciliation and creativity.
- A positive person is an adult who thinks that others are as important as she or he is.
- He or she always remains his or her usual natural self, and an incorrigible optimist.
- They don't waste their energy defending their points of view, nurturing anger and hurtfulness.
- Positive thinking, feeling and actions protect and promote good health. ■

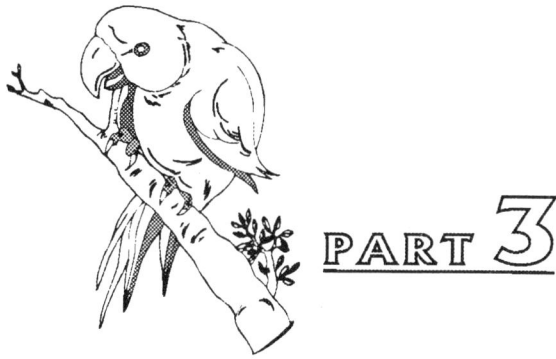

PART 3

NATURE CURES

"He's the best physician that knows the worthlessness of the most medicines."

Franklin

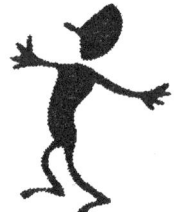

COMMON NATURE CURE CHART FOR GOOD HEALTH

6 a.m.

Upon rising from bed, three glasses of pure lukewarm water with one tablespoonful of honey and juice of half a lemon.

6 a.m.- 6.45 a.m.

Brisk morning walk for 40 minutes in clean and green environment with deep breathing or yogic exercises. Chew 5-7 holy basil (*Tulsi*) leaves before, during or after the walk or exercise.

6.45 a.m.

Green Water (*GW*) at least twice a day—pure water filled in green coloured bottle up to $3/4^{th}$ and sun charged for minimum of 8 hours.

7.30 a.m.

Amla Water (*AW*)—10-12 pieces of fresh/dried clean *amla* in a glass of water soaked overnight.

8.30 a.m.

Breakfast 10-12 raisins *(munnakka* or *kismish)*, 3 figs *(anjir)* soaked overnight and seasonal fruits.

12.00-1 p.m.

Lunch 50% salad, 2-3 chapatis (made from whole wheat mixed with black gram and soyabean in the ratio 10:2:1), boiled or steamed vegetables, green *chutney*/pickles (made of *amla* (Indian gooseberry), *pudina* (mint) and *dhania* (coriander leaves).

Alternatively, sprouts with dates, *munakka* and honey.

5 p.m.

Fresh fruit juice one glass or one seasonal fruit.

6-6.30 p.m.

GW or AW

7.00-8 p.m.

Dinner 50% salad and fruit and rest 50% same as lunch (Preceded or followed by 30 minutes walk).

Other Tips

- If constipated, lukewarm neem or lemon water enema.
- Oil massage for 40 minutes in the morning sun once or twice a week.

- Dry massage for 15 minutes every day before bath.
- Steam bath once or twice a week.
- At least 7 hours of sleep at night (9.30 p.m.-5 a.m.).
- Drinking a total of 14 glasses of water or fluids (3 litres) every day. (Including lemon, amla, green water, fruit juice, soup, butter milk, etc.)
- Avoid milk products (except butter milk and yoghurt), sweets, *maida* products, salts, pickles, *paan* masala, tobacco, drugs, soft drinks, white polished rice, tea, coffee, alcohol, smoking, processed foods, fried foods, *chaats,* flesh foods and other stimulants.
- Pray, meditate and think positive. This is a common chart and preventive in nature. It may be modified in case of some diseases in consultation with a naturopath. For instance, in case of some skin problems like vitiligo, citrus food is excluded and in case of hepatic disorders, milk is added. While taking food, it should be kept in mind that *morning is the time for elimination, day for appropriation* and *night for assimilation.* Because of this reason, dinner must be over by 8 p.m. ■

SOME COMMON DISORDERS AND NATURAL REMEDIES

RHEUMATOLOGICAL DISORDERS

RHEUMATOLOGICAL DISORDERS are as common as cold. There are more than 100 types such as arthritis, gout, spondylosis, etc. Of these, arthritis alone is of 96 types. These are mostly problems of the joints and can be prevented with positive lifestyles, exercise and modified food habits. Nature has created a wonderful, architectural arrangement of bones, muscles and joints to help and support the human body, its internal organs, and to provide agility and mobility. The joints are provided with fibrous capsules of connective tissues which secrete fluids to lubricate the moving parts. Ligaments surrounding the joint help keep the movement within safe limits.

Osteo Arthritis

It is a degenerative or wear and tear disease of the joints

---

*The remedies are suggestive and to be followed in consultation with a qualified naturopath.

common in elderly people. It affects large weight bearing joints like knees, hips and also spine. Obese people are more vulnerable to this. The disease causes joint stiffness, pain, swelling and limitation of motion. Pain increases with motion and decreases with rest.

Treatment Tips

The objective of treatment is to relieve pain, prevent recurrence and disability.

- Follow CNCC and start with gentle massage with red oil and exercise of joints. Take a weight reducing diet. It is better to start with a short fast.
- Hot and cold fomentation to affected joints.
- Regular exercise to improve muscle tone.
- Cold and hot compress in the affected area to treat localized inflammation and pain.
- Hot mud pack on the affected parts.
- Alkaline diet. Vegetables like cabbage, carrot, cucumber, lettuce, onion, radishes and tomatoes as raw salads. Exclude all flesh foods.
- Cooked or boiled vegetables grown organically may include beet, cauliflower, carrot, brinjal, mushroom, green peas, beans, spinach, turnips, tomato, etc
- Cut down sugar consumption to one teaspoonful a day.
- In severe cases, patients may be put on raw vegetable juice

therapy for a week. Alkaline action of raw juice dissolves deposits around the joints. Raw potato juice is also effective.

- Water of fenugreek seeds soaked overnight to be taken early morning on empty stomach. Water kept overnight in copper container also helps.

- Green gram soups mixed with powdered fenugreek seeds.

- Neutral hip-bath with Epsom salts for 15-20 minutes.

- Lots of salads and roughage fruits to avoid constipation. *Karela* juice (bitter gourd) clears the bowels.

- *Amla,* honey, lemon green water also help.

- To prevent the leaching of calcium from bones take potassium-foods like—amaranth leaves, tomatoes, banana, moong dal, brinjal, yogurt and magnesium-rich food like beans, whole grains, millets, nuts and mangoes.

- Helpful yogic asanas are: *Bhujangasana, shavasana, naukasan* and *pawan muktasan.* Walking two kilometer a day increases bone mineral density.

- Lukewarm enema for a few days. Cold baths to be avoided.

- Avoid meat, fish, pulses, high protein diet, sprouts, coffee, tea, chocolate, alcohol.

- Patients with high ESR, uric acid or high blood sugar level may take a longer period in getting relief.

- Avoid living in dark houses, crowded places, treeless areas and places that lack sunshine.

Rheumatoid Arthritis

It affects all joints in the body and damages connective tissues and organs including heart and lungs. Most commonly affected joints are those of the fingers, base of toes, wrists, knees, ankles, shoulders, hips and elbows. Women are three times more vulnerable than men.

Treatment Tips

- CNCC
- Fill small plastic bags with ice and seal them—hold one over and one under each painful knee for 10-15 minutes every 3-4 hours.
- Frequent warm water baths.
- Daily hot foot bath.
- Cold pack to inflamed joints.
- Hot mud pack to affected joints.
- Vegetable or raw potato juice and garlic juice with water every three hours.
- Grapes and raisins, raw goat milk.
- Brown rice or whole wheat bread.
- Fenugreek water soaked overnight.
- Acupressure.
- Regular cleansing of bowels.

- Adequate rest.

Spondylitis

It is an inflammatory disorder of the spinal cord causing stiffness and rigidity in areas close to the spine.

Treatment Tips

- CNCC
- Apply RICE principle:

    R—Rest for the painful area.

    I—Ice cold packs at repeated intervals.

    C—Cold compresses frequently.

    E—Elevation of affected area to help movement of accumulated blood to other areas.

- Gentle massage with hot and cold fomentation.
- Accupressure.
- Regular back bending exercises.
- Avoid lifting of weight or sudden jerks.

Gout

This is a form of arthritis caused by deposition of monosodium urate crystals in joints. Ninety per cent of gout patients comprise men over fifty years. It affects peripheral joints and mostly the toes.

Treatment Tips

- CNCC
- Treatment specifically suggested for arthritis.
- Acupressure.

Frozen Shoulder

Treatment Tips

- CNCC
- Gentle massage followed by hot and cold fomentation.
- Cold pack for one hour at night regularly.
- Physiotherapy and movement of shoulder joints in all directions.
- Acupressure.

In all rheumatic disorders, foods rich in vitamin A,C, & D should be taken. Diet should include plenty of vegetables, dates and figs, garlic, fenugreek, a pinch of *hing* (asafoetida). Exclude vinegar, white sugar, calcium foods, cakes, biscuits, cream, all nuts including almond and non-vegetarian foods. Take plenty of water.

RESPIRATORY DISORDERS

Asthma

It is a Greek word meaning 'Panting or short drawn breath'. Asthma is a chronic pulmonary disease characterized by hyper responsiveness to various stimuli, resulting in widespread narrowing of airways. Persons with asthma are troubled by frequent attacks of breathlessness.

Treatment Tips

Unfortunately, modern medicine hardly offers a cure for asthma. The following naturopathic ways are very effective:

- CNCC, but avoid vigorous exercises.
- Juice fast for a few days.
- Regular enema to clean the colon and prevent autointoxication.
- Mud packs on the abdomen.
- Wet packs on the chest to relieve lung congestion.
- Patient should be helped to perspire through steam bath (alternate days), hot foot bath, hot hip bath and sun bath.
- Avoid or reduce intake of acid forming foods (carbohydrates, fats and proteins).
- Take plenty of alkaline foods like fresh fruit and green vegetables. Apple, carrot and cabbage juice also help.
- Phlegm producing foods like sugar, rice, curds, lentils, fried and heavy foods should be avoided.
- One tablespoon of garlic juice mixed with honey and a glass of water in the morning followed half an hour later with half cup of bitter gourd juice.

- Steam inhalation, sauna bath.

- Fruit for breakfast, boiled/steamed vegetables, salad and whole wheat bread for lunch and dinner; sun dried fruits like figs, dates, apricot, pear may be added to breakfast.

- Take early dinner and avoid heavy meals.

- Salt intake must be reduced to 2 grams a day.

- All aluminium cooking vessels to be discarded.

- *Jalneti* and *Yogasanas (Bhujangasana, Dhanurasana, Ardhamatsyenderasana, Puschimottanasana, Sarvangasana, Shavasana).*

- Keep all the things you are allergic to at a distance.

- Keep away from pollen, dogs, cats and horses, feathers in pillows and quilts, aspirin and dispirin.

Bronchitis

This breathing disorder is caused by the inflammation of the mucous membrane lining and bronchial tube within the chest. Airway infection is the primary mechanism of airway obstruction. The problem is endemic to cold and damp climates but is also found in other climates. High fever, deep chest cough, difficulty in breathing, hoarseness in throat, pain in chest and loss of appetite are common symptoms. Excessive smokers and people with wrong food habits are more prone to this problem.

Treatment Tips

- CNCC.

- One tablespoon of onion juice in the morning.

- Fasting on orange juice mixed (with 50 per cent water) every two hours for two days.

- Followed by all fruit diet for another two days.

- Then follow the diet as mentioned in CNCC.

- Water mixed with turmeric powder twice a day on empty stomach; also radish juice with water at least twice a day.

- Boiled concoction of ginger, black pepper and holy basil (*Tulsi*), three times a day.

- Steam inhalation, fomentation of upper and middle back.

- A hot Epsom salt bath at least three times a week (body to be immersed in bath for 20 minutes).

- Yogic *Kriyas*, chest physiotherapy, hot foot bath, *Jalneti* and simple *Pranayama*.

- Breathing exercise includes taking slow and deep breath and exhaling slowly and completely with lips pursed; apply gentle pressure on upper abdomen to squeeze the remaining air from lungs—repeat 20 times, thrice a day.

- Avoid soft drinks, refrigerated food, tea, coffee, condiments, pickles, flesh foods.

Sinusitis

Sinuses are empty spaces in the skull area connected with the nasal passage. So any infection in nose or throat may infect the sinuses. Accumulation of secretions in sinus area leads to heaviness in head, nasal obstruction, discharge and pain, lack of appetite, toothache and low fever.

Treatment Tips

- CNCC with preference for alkaline diet rich in vitamin A.
- Enema for 3 days and juice fasting for 3 days (carrot, beet or cucumber)
- Garlic and onion juice, one tablespoon, thrice daily.
- Steam inhalation, steam bath and massage over sinus area.
- Hot foot bath and *Jalneti*.
- Avoid sugar, salt, *maida* products, rice, cakes and candies.
- Plenty of sleep, rest and fresh air.

Common Cold, Cough, Tonsillitis

Treatment Tips

- CNCC
- Drink plenty of warm water and orange or yellow fruit juice.
- Breathe clean, non-smoky air; eat carrots and dark green vegetables and soups.
- In cases of sore throat, saline gargling every 4 hours.
- Hot foot bath, steam bath, steam inhalation.
- Combine 30 gms sliced ginger, one broken cinnamon stick,

one tsp. coriander seeds, six tulsi leaves, three cloves, one slice of lemon and 2 glass full of water. Simmer for 20 minutes, strain and drink a hot cup full every 3 hours.

- Or take ginger, *tulsi* juice with honey every 3 hours.
- Throat pack for tonsillitis.
- Cough and cold among children may develop into pneumonia. Breast feeding is the best preventive against it.

GASTRO-INTESTINAL DISORDERS

These disorders are responsible for most of our health problems. They arise out of our eating habits and faulty lifestyle. Gastritis, constipation, diabetes, indigestion, peptic ulcer, diarrhea and liver disorders are the consequences.

Gastritis

It is caused by an inflammation of the stomach lining. Lack of fluid intake and constipation aggravate it. Over-eating, eating cold combinations of foods, excessive intake of tea, coffee or alcoholic drinks contribute to gastritis. The main symptoms are loss of appetite, nausea, vomiting, and headache.

Treatment Tips

- CNCC and fasting for 2/3 days on fruit juices.
- Followed by all fruit diet for 3 days.
- Food to be swallowed after vigorous mastication.
- One apple at bed time.

- Hot compress on empty stomach.
- Green coconut water is an excellent food remedy.
- Avoid nicotine, condiments, chillies, fresh foods, pickles, strong tea, coffee, pastries, cakes and fried foods.

Constipation

It is a very common disorder of the digestive tract. In this condition bowels do not clear easily. As a result, toxins are produced and these enter into blood stream, causing various types of diseases. Common symptoms are foul breath, coated tongue, ulcers in the mouth, fullness in abdomen, nausea, headache, loss of appetite, acidity, heart burn, insomnia, fissure, piles, etc. Eating disorder is the main culprit in constipation.

Treatment Tips

- CNCC plus enema and exclusive fruit diet for five days.
- *Amla* water and bitter gourd juice alternately.
- Eat lot of salad, green and leafy vegetables, fibre foods and fruit. Take food only when hungry.
- Figs, raisins (soaked overnight) and dates for breakfast.
- Intermittent drinking of warm water with lime juice with half teaspoon of salt.
- A teaspoonful of almond oil mixed with a glass of warm milk before going to bed. Alternatively two tablespoons of Isabgol powder in a glass of water followed by another glass of water before going to bed.

- Alternatively *Bael* fruit or powder (two tablespoons) mixed with water, two hours before food.
- Avoid white flour, white rice, bread, pulses, cakes, pastries, all milk products, cheese, flesh foods and hard boiled eggs.
- Sun charged green water before going to bed.
- Alternate hot and cold hip bath.
- *Bhujangasana, Dhanurasana, Halasana, Puschimotanasana, Ardhamatsyendrasana.*

Indigestion, dyspepsia

It is caused by over-eating, improper eating or eating too rapidly, eating without hunger, eating frequently and/or heavy foods. Symptoms of indigestion are loss of appetite, nausea, vomiting, excessive wind or gas, heartburn, acidity and abdominal pain.

Treatment Tips

- CNCC plus enema and an all-fruit diet for a few days.
- Followed by lightly cooked or steamed vegetables, juicy fruit and butter milk for a week.
- One teaspoon of ginger juice, fresh lime, mint juice mixed with one teaspoon of honey after meals.
- Lemon juice with water and a pinch of salt every three hours.
- Orange juice twice a day, follow the chapter on Food Friends.
- Avoid eating and drinking together.

- Avoid eating to a full stomach, miss a meal until appetite returns.

- Masticate food properly, avoid eating when too tired or in tension.

- *Vajrasana* after lunch and dinner.

- *Kunjal.*

- Alternate hot & cold hip bath in the evening.

- Aniseed or *saunf* is ideal for expelling wind, gas and helping digestion. One teaspoon in a cup of boiling water covered overnight and to be taken in the morning with honey.

- Early dinner (7.30 p.m.) followed by a walk for 30 minutes.

Diarrhoea

Frequent passage of loose or watery stool is called diarrhea. It causes rapid dehydration. Millions of children die every year due to diarrhea. Poor hygiene, lack of clean drinking water and wrong food habits are the main causes.

Treatment Tips

- It can be prevented by keeping food and water clean, using latrines and washing hands properly every time before taking food.

- Avoid salads until full recovery.

- Plenty of boiled, warm water should be taken to replace loss of fluids.

- Oral Rehydration Solution (ORS) should be administered to treat dehydration.

- Grind two leaves of *Hemkedar* or *Patharchata* with seven black peppers mixed with one cup of water twice a day taken at 15 minutes interval; mint leaves ground with black pepper also help.

- After acute symptoms are over, pomegranate fruit juice and steamed raw banana or vegetables can be taken.

- Butter milk is an effective remedy as it fights germs and bacteria. Can be taken 3-4 times a day with a pinch of salt.

Dysentery

It is caused by infection of the large intestine and spreads due to unhygienic sanitary conditions. The two organisms responsible for it are protozoa and bacilli. The former causes amoebic dysentery and the latter, bacillary dysentery. Of these, the amoebic is more difficult to treat. Both the types are characterized by regular liquid or semi liquid stools, mucous & blood, inflammation, ulceration of bowel and colic pain. The main culprit in dysentery is dietary indiscretion.

Treatment Tips

- Low pressure enema.
- Orange juice and water fasting.
- Alternatively, live on butter milk till acute symptoms alleviated.

- Small doses of castor oil to remove offensive matter from the system and for lubrication of ulcerated surface.

- Amoeba parasite to be eliminated through cold hip bath, mud pack.

- *Bael* fruit (stone apple) mixed with water and jaggery twice a day.

- Rice mixed with curd, steamed vegetables, sprouts, fresh and ripe fruits may be taken.

- Regular exercise.

Peptic Ulcer

An open sore in the mucous membrance is known as ulcer. The ulcer located in the stomach or duodenum is called peptic ulcer. This is caused by an increase in hydrochloric acid in stomach. A common symptom is severe pain in the abdomen. Over-eating, heavy or highly spiced foods, coffee, alcohol, smoking, stress and tension are the main causative factors. Naturopaths call peptic ulcer a result of *hurry, worry and curry*. It is more common in people with blood group 'O' and with respiratory diseases.

Treatment Tips

- CNCC plus controlled and plain diet and rest to the affected organ; plain water enema if constipated.

- In the morning take 50 gram raisins soaked overnight along with water.

- Milk, butter milk, fruits and steamed vegetable diet; chew well before eating.

- In an advanced stage, banana and milk diet is very beneficial.
- Boiled cabbage water twice a day supplemented with raw vegetable juices or tender coconut water; avoid white and polished rice, chilly, spices, nuts, steaming hot drinks.
- Avoid eating when tired or depressed or not hungry.
- When pain is severe, take frequent, short light foods.
- Cold water bath twice a day and hot and cold hip baths.
- Mud pack on empty stomach and hot pack in case of abdominal pain.
- Avoid salty food and any food that causes discomfort; keep the stomach light.
- Avoid painkillers, aspirins and anti-inflammatory drugs.
- Regular exercise, *vajrasana, puschimottanasana, Jalneti* and *Pranayama*.
- Good quality sleep is always beneficial as it heals the ulcer faster.

LIVER DISORDERS

Liver is one of the most critical organs in the body involved in the metabolism and storage of nutrients. It is located on the right side of the abdomen under the diaphragm and works like a chemical laboratory. Its main function is secretion of bile which is essential for digestion of fats. Liver also produces enzymes which control the chemical process in the body. Excessive eating, poor nutrition, bad food, alcohol consumption, drugs, overloading and viral infections causes liver damage. In Hepatitis Naturopathy helps in regenerating of the liver tissue through dietary treatment to prevent further damage.

Treatment Tips

- Warm water enema.
- CNCC plus initial liver cleaning with juice fast for three days.
- Beets, lemon, papaya and grape juice are the best.
- Followed by fruit and milk diet for one week.
- Sugarcane juice, cabbage juice, radish juice and carrot juice are very useful.
- Raw nuts, almonds, home made cheese, sprouts and steamed vegetables like papaya, bitter gourd, beets, baked potato may follow the milk and fruit diet. Salt, sugar to be reduced.
- Potassium-rich vegetables and fruits are recommended to improve biliary tract functions – these are dried apricot, dates, peaches, baked potatoes, cabbage, turnip, oranges, bananas raisins, fig, fresh cucumbers etc.
- Add tender neem leaves, flowers to your diet at least twice a week.
- Application of alternate compress to liver area.
- *Pranayama*, deep breathing twice every day.
- Exclude alcohol completely.

- Plenty of liquids, vegetable soups and complete bed rest in case of *jaundice* or hepatitis.

- Exclude all fats, fried foods, smoked foods, cakes, creams, pulses, legumes and all kinds of meat.

- Instead of full meals, take frequent fractional meals every 3-4 hours.

- In case of Hepatitis a low volume high caloric diet is needed to maintain weight and ensure maximum protein utilization.

- An intake of 1 to 2 gm protein per kg of body weight is recommended. Sodium is restricted to 2 gm a day.

- Mud packs, mineral water drinks and sulphide mineral bath diminish inflammation.

URINARY DISORDERS

The urinary tract is a very important part of the body consisting of kidney, ureter, bladder and urethra. Nature has provided each individual with two kidneys, each one of which has one million nephrons or filtering units. If CNCC is properly followed many urinary disorders could be prevented.

Kidney Stone & Urinary Tract Infection

It is a common urinary disorder. Stones are formed in the kidney or urinary tract from chemicals in the urine like uric acid, calcium, oxalic acid and phosphorus. Such stones cause severe pain when they attempt to pass down the ureter on their way to the bladder. Painful, scanty urination, nausea and vomiting are some of the symptoms.

Treatment Tips

- CNCC minus lemon; avoid foods that irritate kidney like condiments, alcohol, pickles etc.
- Sufficient fluid intake to prevent urine concentration.
- Proper genital hygiene; avoid genital contact with infected things.
- Maintain ideal body weight and take a low protein diet.
- *Avoid* high intake of milk, alkali or Vitamin D.
- *Avoid* whole wheat flour, Bengal gram, soyabeans, spinach, almonds, coconut, tomato, beet and radish.
- Food should consist of fresh green peas, pumpkin, cauliflower, cabbage, turnips, beans, etc.
- Take fruits like watermelon, grapes and apple. Paste of pomegranate seeds also helps.
- For all kidney and bladder troubles, slowly boil 75 mg of fresh bean pods in seven litres of water for three hour, filter the liquid, allow it to cool for six hours and give a glassful every two hours to the patient with the kidney problem.
- For kidney stones, basil juice with honey may be taken for six months.
- Hot enema followed by hot bath; *Bhujangasana, Halasana, Dhanurasana* are beneficial.
- Dietary calcium should not exceed 800-1000 mg.
- Kidney stones are 'what you eat' and therefore diet modification is very important.

Prostate Disorders

Prostate is a male gland situated at the base of urinary bladder to facilitate passage of urine. It also plays an important role in sexual life. Mostly men above 50 are prone to prostate related disorders like inflammation of the prostate gland, difficulty in passing urine, increased urine frequency during sleep at night, pain in the hips or lower back. Prolonged sitting, constipation, excessive sexual excitement adversely effect the prostate gland. Surgery is needed as a last resort.

Treatment Tips

- As a preventive measure keep the bladder healthy. Relieve yourself every 2/3 hours.
- *Avoid* antihistamines, cough syrups, antispasmodics, antidepressants, indiscriminate drug use.
- CNCC minus all solid foods for three days followed by all fruit diet for three days when prostate is detected.
- Subsist on water every hour when awake, mixed with one tsp of tulsi juice.
- *Avoid* sexual excesses alcohol.
- Enema once a day to clear bowels if constipated.
- Follow a plain light diet from the fourth day onwards. Dinner should consist of steam cooked vegetables with good sources of selenium like beans, pulses and leafy vegetables.
- Add pumpkin seeds to the diet and exclude spices, flesh foods, fried foods, sauces, condiments, cheese, potato, brinjal, radish, salt, pepper and anything sour or irritating.

- Regular drinking of honey water is the best natural preventive measure.
- Eat more fibre to avaoid constipation.
- Add figs, white onion, cabbage, cucumbers, cauliflower to your diet to make up silicon deficiency.
- Green and yellow vegetables, raw juice mixture, cucumber are very useful.
- Eating lots of broccoli helps prevent prostate cancer.
- Foods grown in selenium rich soil is also a very good preventive against lung, colon and prostate cancers.
- Avoid sitting for more than 45 minutes at a time.
- Hot and cold application on and around prostate gland helps.
- Alternate hot and cold baths (10 min : 1 minute) has also been found to be effective.

ANORECTAL DISORDERS

Piles, Fissure and Fistula comprise the main anorectal problems. They arise from faulty eating habits and incorrect lifestyles. All these disorders can be prevented through modification of food and work habits.

Piles

Its other name is haemorrhoids. It is an inflamed condition of the veins in or around the rectum. External pile give lot of pain and internal pile discharges dark blood. The patient is unable to sit on account of pain and discomfort. The main cause is chronic constipation and other bowel disorders.

Treatment Tips

- All-fruit diet for three days.
- CNCC with added emphasis on fibrous and roughage foods consisting of fruit, vegetables, wheat bran and unpolished rice.
- Completely avoid spicy, fatty, fried and calorie rich foods.
- A minimum of 15 glasses of liquids a day.
- Follow the treatment suggested for constipation.
- Mud pack, cold and warm hip bath, brish walk and yoga.
- Ensure anorectal hygiene and apply til, castor or coconut oil to lubricate the anal area.

Fissure and Fistula

It is a cut in or around anal canal and mucus membrane mostly on account of straining while passing stool during chronic dysentery and severe constipation. In Fistula, the rectum or anal canal gets infected forming a tunnel through which pus dribbles. Fissure also may lead to Fistula. It is very painful and generally treated with surgery. Even after surgery, fistula is notorious for recurrence. Such recurrence could be prevented if the dietary discipline suggested for piles is strictly followed. For Fissure, curing constipation and applying hot and cold pack to the anal area are of great help. Seitz bath in warm water every day for 30 minutes is beneficial for all types of Anorectal disorders. Strict adherence to CNCC helps prevention of fissure and fistula.

DIABETES

It is a metabolic disorder caused by lack of a digestive hormone called insulin, and inability of the body to use the available insulin. Diabetes makes treatment of other diseases complicated. It is also linked to loss of brain tissue, dementia and Alzheimer's disease. Two characteristic symptoms are:

(i) Copious urination, and

(ii) Glucose in the urine.

A diabetic person often feels hungry, thirsty and gets easily tired. Over consumption of sugar, refined carbohydrates, proteins and fats, obesity, lack of physical exercise and stress contribute to diabetes. It may also be hereditary.

Treatment Tips

- CNCC minus honey water plus one teaspoonful of broken fenugreek (*methi*) seeds with water in the morning.
- Followed half an hour later by bitter gourd (four or five nos.) juice every morning on an empty stomach.
- Consumption of not more than 1500 calories a day (900 carbohydrates, 350 fats, 250 proteins) : High fibre and high carbohydrate diet.
- Exclude sugar, honey, jam, chocolates, sweets, alcohol, white rice and processed foods.
- Foods including vegetables which can be taken are cabbage, tomato, radish, carrots, green peas, beet, onion, garlic muschroom, spinach, string beans, whole wheat bread, boiled potato (up to 100 gm), and curd.

- Fresh fruit, raw foods and sprouts are very good as they stimulate insulin production.
- Avoid worry, stress and strain.
- Light exercises, *Bhujangasana, Paschimottanasana, Halasana, Ardhmatsyendrasana, Jalneti, Kunjal.*
- For sedentary person, at least 4-5 kilometres of walk either in the morning or evening, or both times.

OBESITY

A person with a weight 20 per cent more than normal is an obese person. Over-eating is the main cause of obesity. Napoleon's life was shortened because of over-eating and obesity although he was a man of tremendous energy. More people in world die of over-eating than starvation. When one eats more calories than one uses, the extra calories give you one extra pound of weight. And even if you eat less, you can still gain extra weight if you are physically inactive. Obesity is also common in affluent societies. Obese people fall prey to a number of diseases, i.e., diabetes, high blood pressure, heart ailments, gall bladder stones, arthritis, inflated tummy and liver complications. Obesity can reduce one's lifespan by 30 per cent.

Treatment Tips

- Complete juice and water fasting for five days followed by CNCC eating plan and plain water enema.
- Eat when really hungry and not when attracted by food; stop eating when satisfied.

- Follow 4-4-2-2 formula, i.e. four servings of fruit and vegetables, two servings of cereals and other grain products, two servings of butter milk every day; juice fast for three days followed by all fruit diet for another three days—once in every two months until normal weight is restored.

- Those who find juice fast difficult, can have soup fast, butter milk or barley water fast.

- Take fruit for breakfast, boiled green vegetables for lunch and dinner with plenty of salads.

- Avoid oil, butter, cheese, ghee, chocolates, cream, fried foods, gravy, candy, cake, potatoes, puddings, alcoholic drinks, flesh foods, tea, coffee, smoking.

- Chew food to pulp before swallowing.

- Do not eat when tired, angry or worried.

- Another effective remedy is to live on honey-lime juice water for two days, followed by lemon juice water fast for one day, once in every fortnight.

- Morning, evening brisk walks for 45 minutes or until one gets tired, *Sarvangasana, Halasana, Dhanuransana, Chakrasana, Puschimottanasana, Vajrasana* help fight obesity.

HIGH BLOOD PRESSURE

The total volume of blood forms about one-twelfth of the weight of the body or about 5 litres. When blood exerts pressure against the walls of the arteries, it is called blood pressure. This is essential for circulation, exchange of nutrients and waste products and also for filtering and purification of blood in the kidneys and lungs. Blood pressure increases when the heart contracts, and decreases when the heart expands. These two pressures are *considered normal* if they are *90-140 mm Hg and 70-90 mm Hg respectively. When this normal ratio is exceeded it is called high blood pressure* or hypertension.

High blood pressure may remain hidden without warning and manifest suddenly in the form of stroke or heart attack. Symptoms may appear in the form of pain in the back of head, neck, dizziness, and pain in the limbs, fatigue, nervous tension, frequent urination. Cholesterol, diabetes, kidney problems, defective heart and faulty lifestyle are the **main causes**. An obese, negative, aggressive, ill tempered, impatient, ambitious person with an irregular, hurried and worried lifestyle is more vulnerable to high blood pressure than others. Heredity is also one of the causes.

Treatment Tips

- CNCC with added emphasis on regular walk and jogging.
- Maintain ideal body weight.
- Learn to relax, slow down the pace of life.
- Eat less fat, less salt, less sugar and observe one fat-salt-sugarless day in a week.
- Abandon alcohol and smoking altogether.
- A well balanced routine of correct diet consisting of fresh fruit and vegetables; add garlic.
- Try to live on a fruit diet for at least three days (three times at five hourly intervals); return to normal diet gradually.

- One tablespoon of amla juice with honey in the morning followed by *ashgourd* juice—one cup after 30 minutes. Inhalation of almond oil and taking one teaspoon of almond oil with a cup of warm cow milk at bedtime is very useful.

- Fruits like apple, cucumber, melon, pineapple, papaya and *bathua* (goosefoot), coriander and mint leaves are good both for heart and blood pressure.

- Neutral bath for 45 minutes with cold compress on the head is very helpful.

- Cold water enema when the BP becomes high.

- *Shavasana, Vajrasana, Makarasana* and meditation.

- A positive attitude, cheerful and contented mind.

HEART DISORDERS

Heart is like a *pump house* that supplies blood to all parts of the body. Blood carries oxygen to brain and other parts. Without oxygen, body cells stop working. An adult heart beats 70 times a minute and this speed also changes in response to needs. It pounds faster during exercise, lovemaking, fear, grief and anger. When the arteries carrying blood get clogged or narrowed by fat or calcium deposits, heart problems begin. Eventually, it leads to coronary malfunction and heart attacks. Obesity, diabetes, blood pressure, smoking, stress, faulty food habits and wrong lifestyle increase the risk of heart disorder. The effect of fat and cholesterol on heart has already been discussed. *The following tips are additional.*

Treatment Tips

- Religiously follow the CNCC.

- Risk to heart can be prevented and reduced through regular exercise and by eating simple carbohydrates. Legs are called the second heart; the more they are used, the less the fear for heart and lungs.

- A glass of *amla* water in the morning—followed by one teaspoon of onion juice with honey is a tonic for the heart.

- Breakfast may consist of fresh fruit or *dalia* or brown bread and yoghurt.

- Eat a variety of grain products especially whole grains.

- Take low calorie, low fat, high fibre food; reduce sugar and salt intake; an early dinner.

- Take sweet fruit after lunch and dinner; avoid dessert.

- Soyabean foods, oat bran, onion, alfalfa, mint, coriander, goosefoot and garlic have properties to prevent cardiovascular complications.

- A glass of fresh fruit juice or coconut water in the afternoon or fresh fruits like apple, orange, pomegranate, pineapple, grapes, orange juice, prevents heart attacks.

- Keep calm, avoid extreme emotions, excitement, arguments.

- Breathing exercises every day to inhale more oxygen from fresh air.

- A stress-free life with proper rest, relaxation and sleep keeps the heart strong and young.

STROKES

It is a kind of brain attack caused by sudden interruption of blood supply, glucose and oxygen, to parts of brain. It has emerged as a leading cause of adult disability and deaths in the world. Yet strokes can be prevented. Some of the signals of stroke are: sudden numbness of face, arm or leg—on one side of the body, sudden confusion, impaired speech, dimness of vision, dizziness, trouble in walking etc.

Preventive Steps:

- Follow tips on heart disorders.
- Control blood pressure, diabetes and cholesterol if any.
- Avoid smoking, alcohol, fats and obesity.
- Eat plenty of fruits and vegetables—it unblocks cholesterol.
- Cut sodium, go for potassium rich foods like banana, orange, almonds, apricot, cooked spinach, sweet potato, skimmed milk.
- Keep active and improve your circulation, cardio-vascular system, walking, jogging, cycling, swimming, dancing at least five times a week.
- Avoid fried stuff, milk products, chocolates, French fries, pastries.
- Avoid back-to-back work schedules.
- Yoga, meditation, relaxation exercises.
- Get adequate sleep, think positive.
- Have regular medical check-ups.

CANCER

Cancer is the second most common cause of death in the world next to heart disease. The word cancer is derived from the Latin word 'carcinoma' which means crab. There are more than 100 types of cancer, and in India every year more than 6,00,000 people die of disease.

Cancer is caused by an abnormal and uncontrolled division of cells that refuse to stop multiplying. They do not remain confined to any part of the body and travel by blood and lymph channels. Manifestations of cancer may include:

(i) A lump or hard area in the breast

(ii) A change in wart or mole

(iii) Persistent change in bowel habits

(iv) Non-injury bleeding

(v) An ulcer that refuses to heal

(vi) Unexplained loss of weight and appetite

(vii) Unexplained low grade fever

If detected early, most of the cancers can be cured. Yet the best thing is to prevent occurrence through a regulated and disciplined living. Dietary habits and lifestyle changes can prolong life once the cancerous growth is removed.

Treatment Tips

- Thorough cleaning of the system by enema, *Kunjal, Jalneti,* and juice fasting for one week.

- Consume two tender *neem* and *tulsi* (holy basil) leaves everyday in the morning on empty stomach.

- All the organs of elimination, i.e., liver, kidney, lungs, bowels and skin need to be revitalized. For instance, a diet free from animal protein can rejuvenate the liver faster. High fibre diet reactivates bowels. *Pranayama* vitalizes lungs. Adequate intake of fluids and juices strengthens the kidney. A fruit diet for a week helps all vital parts.

- Alternate drinking of carrot juice and wheat grass juice have proved to be very effective. This furnishes the body with live minerals, vitamins and trace elements.

- Some naturopaths recommend grape cure. After a two day short fast the patient is kept on a grape fruit diet—every two hours from 8 a.m. to 8 p.m. There are instances when people have recovered from early stages of breast cancer by living on raw potato juice, carrot juice, cabbage and garlic juice for 40 days under supervision of a qualified naturopath.

- Organically grown citrus fruits, green and yellow vegetables, melon, dry fruits are good agents in preventing cancer. Incidence of cancer is reported to be much less in vegetarian societies.

- Eating vegetables from the cruciferous family, like broccoli and cabbage are known to deduce cancer risks.

- Two or three almonds, soaked and peeled, taken regularly at breakfast, act as a good preventive.

- In northern China, where garlic and onion are abundantly produced, incidence of stomach cancer is the lowest.

◘ High beta carotene of fresh apricots and henzaldehyde in figs are good cancer fighters with preventive and curative properties.

◘ Avoid smoking, tobacco chewing, alcohol, *maida* products, processed, canned, salted, oily, spiced foods and foods grown with the help of chemical fertilizers and pesticides. Avoid cooking in aluminium vessels.

◘ Live and work in a relatively pollution free environment, walk one hour every day along with deep breathing; take adequate rest and don't be afraid.

◘ Following CNCC steadfastly can prevent the risk of cancer and many other difficult diseases.

PYORRHOEA AND TOOTHACHE

This is a disease of the teeth socket. It effects the membrance around the teeth root, weakens the teeth, forms pus and attacks the gum, leading to loss of teeth. About half of our adult population suffers from this disease. It is primarily caused by bacterial activity, lack of dental hygiene, wrong eating habits and acidosis. Pyorrhoea may also be hereditary.

Treatment Tips

◘ Clean the bowels with warm water enema daily.

◘ Begin with a short juice fast for three days (fresh carrot or orange and water) at two hourly intervals from 8 a.m. to 9 p.m.

◘ GW and AW twice daily.

- Followed by fresh fruit diet for another three days (one type of fruit at a time).
- Followed by a normal diet as prescribed in the CNCC.
- Exclude all refined and processed foods, condiments, sugar, chocolates, ice cream, sauces, tea, coffee and flesh foods.
- Tooth enamel cannot be replaced by body and needs to be protected by regular brushing; say no to sticky food, cola and tea and wash mouth after every cup of milk or liquid food.
- Boil one part of sesame seeds with three parts water until reduced to half. Cool and apply directly to the tooth. Sesame contains seven pain relieving compounds.
- Mastication of an onion a day protects against a number of tooth disorders.
- Raw spinach juice, mint lemon and lime are also known to be useful as they strengthen the gums and teeth.
- Eating whole wheat *chappati,* chewing and masticating hard and fibrous foods also help.
- Daily brushing of teeth in the morning, after meals, dry friction, hip bath, hot Epsom bath. Daily brushing of teeth with *Neem* or *Karanj* twigs has been found very useful.
- For teeth sensitive to hot, cold, sweet, sour and chewing, keep warm saline water in mouth for five minutes, three times a day.
- Keep one clove in the mouth overnight for a month. For acute

toothache dab some clove oil on a cotton bud and apply directly to the aching tooth (it is analgesic and anaesthetic).

- Apply paste of salt, mustard oil and turmeric powder.

HEADACHE AND MIGRAINE

Headache is a term used for discomfort or pain in the head. Although seventy per cent of patients visiting a doctor complain of headache, majority of headaches are not serious. Headache is nature's signal that there is something wrong somewhere in the body. Some of the common causes are defective eyesight, inflammation of the sinus, sleeplessness, infection, high blood pressure, tumour in the brain, low blood sugar, indigestion, constipation, fatigue, hangover, emotional stress and travel. On the other hand, migraine is a paroxysmal affection causing severe and recurrent headache generally on one side of the head. It is also associated with digestive and liver disorders.

Treatment Tips

- Warm water enema to clean the bowels.
- Follow all tips given on constipation.
- Avoid indigestion; take early dinner.
- Gentle massage on head and neck, shoulder followed by cold pack.
- For migraine, take short juice fast, steam inhalation.
- Drink large quantity of warm water.

- Keep a hot water bag or heating pad on the neck.
- Abdominal pack three hours after dinner; before going to bed, keep a hot water bag or heating pad on the neck.
- Avoid exposure to excessive heat, cold and rain.
- Hot foot bath, steam bath, cold throat pack, cold compress applied on the head and back bring relief.
- Chocolate, cheese, dairy products, citrus fruits, excess tea, coffee can trigger a migraine attack, and therefore, should be avoided.
- Jalneti is very effective in migraine.
- Acupressure, walking, jogging, *Pushchimottanasana*, *Halasana*, *Sarvangasana* and *Shavasana* are also very effective.
- One teaspoon of Triphala powder at bed time with a cup of warm cow milk regularly also help.
- Keep mind as much free as possible from mental worries and anxiety, and have adequate rest and sleep at night.

INSOMNIA

People today are sleeping less and snoring more. Insomnia or sleeplessness is spreading rapidly among those leading a stressful life. Sleep is an everyday requirement of the body for rest, relief and refreshment. The average sleep needs decrease from nine hours at the age of 12 to eight hours at the age of 20, seven hours at forty, six and half hours at sixty to just six hours at the age of eighty and after. Sleep disorders cause obesity, diabetes and heart disease. A recent Japanese study in 2001 reveals that men who slept five hours or less a night were two times more likely to suffer a heart attack than those who slept eight hours. Mental tension is considered the most common cause of sleeplessness. Feelings of anger, frustration, depression, constipation, over-eating, dyspepsia, heavy and late dinner, excessive intake of tea and coffee are also responsible for sleep disorders.

Tips for Improvement

- Exclude sleeping pills and adhere to CNCC food habits.

- Sleep studies indicate that people treated with sleeping pills revert to their dysfunctional sleep pattern within a year of treatment.

- Maintain a regular sleeping schedule: Early to bed, early to rise; banish all worries while going to bed.

- A hot water bath one or two hours before going to bed helps.

- Have an early and light dinner; wear light and loose clothes.

- Before going to bed take a cup of warm milk with one tablespoon of honey, or warm water with honey or take a glass of warm milk with one tablespoon of almond oil before bedtime.

- Avoid quarrels and watching violence on TV at night.

- Lie on your side (not on the back) and relax your muscles and mind; do not try to solve any problem.

- Do not try to sleep; if sleep does not come on its own resort to light reading and listening to low volume music.

- Watch the figures that come behind closed eyelids.
- Try to repeat holy names, or one of God's many names.
- Alternatively, turn your mind to positive and cheerful thoughts or meditate for 6 to 10 minutes to quieten the mind.
- Controlled breathing: Take three deep breaths, hold breath, then repeat; switch off the mind and listen to your own breathing.
- To avoid snoring sleep on your side; use the right pillow that helps keep your airways open. Nasal strips also help.
- Khaskhas/Posta Power—one tsp. with honey at bed time—is a proven remedy.
- Regular exercise, morning and evening walks, walking on green grass.

DEMENTIA

Like body, brain also changes and degenerates. Out of its 100 billion nerve cells, about 100,000 cells die every day—after a certain age. This eventually leads to memory loss. Misplacing eyeglasses, keys, credit cards, forgetting names and places are quite normal in advancing age. Yet when such memory loss affects job skills, performance of familiar tasks, sense of judgment and leads to disorientation of time and place, problems with abstract thinking and change in mood and behavior, impaired language skills, these can be warning signals for Alzheimer's disease for which a medicine is yet to be found. The following nature cure methods have been proved to be effective as a preventive.

Preventive Tips

- Follow the nature cure chart—avoid smoking and drinking.

- Maintain normal blood pressure and optimal level of LDL (bad) and HDL (good) cholesterol and normal blood sugar.

- Follow nature diet given in this book—avoid saturated fat and fatty acids.

- Eat high-fibre foods—avoid processed food and sodium.

- Include almond (soaked and peeled) and figs in your breakfast, massage almond oil on head before going to sleep.

- Exercise regularly—avoid obesity.

- Reduce tension and stress—meditate daily.

- Develop new hobbies, keep reading, learning and applying.

- Go for mentally stimulating, interesting and innovative habits i.e. drawing, painting, sculpture, word puzzles, writing etc.

- A daily intake of foods with folic acid, vitamin B6 and B12.

- Keep the brain alert and body active.

MENSTRUAL DISORDERS

There are various types of menstrual disorders known as Dysmenorrhea (painful menstruation), pre-menstrual tension (PMT), Amenorrhea (absence of menstruation), oligomenorrhoea (infrequent menses), menorrhoea (excessive menstruation), etc.

Treatment Tips

- Daily cleansing of bowels with warm water enema.
- Follow CNCC with an all-fruit diet for four days with focus on *Amla* water.
- Wheat grass juice for one month.
- Beet juice and carrot juice have been found to be very effective.
- Coriander seeds are very beneficial in excessive menstruation.
- One tablespoon of sesame (*Til*) powder with hot water twice daily reduces menstrual pain.
- *Saunf* (Aniseeds) boiled in water and taken twice also helps.
- Avoid eating sour things like pickles and sour curd.
- Avoid keeping stomach empty for a long time.
- Hygiene of the area around the genitalia is very important.
- For heavy bleeding, soak clean multani mitti over night, filter and drink a glassful for one month.

FEVER

Fever is a signal that there is something wrong in the body. In fever, body temperature rises, causing pain and fatigue in the body and distaste in mouth. Acute fever should not be suppressed with antibiotics.

Treatment Tips

- To control high temperature, sponging or bathing with cool (not cold) water.

- Avoid using too many clothes or blankets.
- No solid food till fever subsides.
- Warm water enema in the morning to flush out toxins.
- Plenty of liquids including lemon-honey water, sweet lime juice, green coconut water, vegetable soup.
- *Tulsi* (holy basil) juice with honey (two teaspoons) thrice daily.
- Chest pack and cold compress on the forehead.
- Mud packs three times a day.
- Rubbing the spine with ice to reduce temperature.
- Patient should be kept in a room with cross ventilation for fresh air.
- As the fever subsides, fresh fruit juice, and later on, mono fruit diet for a day before normal diet. ∎

ART OF NATURAL LIVING
BASIC RULES TO REMEMBER

- Remember the six enemies of good health: faulty diet, addiction to stimulants, sedentary lifestyle, mental stress, polluted environment and unsafe drinking water.
- Make it a habit to walk briskly or jog in the morning for at least 40 minutes. Never miss a chance to walk on green grass. It is invigorating.
- Walking in morning sun makes the bone; working in the day maintains the bone and walking in sunset maximizes it.
- Take two/three glasses of water in sitting position upon rising from bed in the morning and thereafter one glass every two hours. Ensure that the water you drink is pure.
- Expose the body to morning sunlight for vitamin D offered free by nature.
- Do not drink water 30 minutes before and within one hour of taking a meal. No water should be taken during meal.
- Brush teeth after every light as well as principal meal, or intake of liquids like milk or tea.
- Pass urine before every meal.

- Eat less and walk more—stroll for half an hour before or after dinner.
- A daily bath in fresh water keeps body free from dirt, odour and infection of the skin.
- Do not eat until you are hungry.
- Lunch should be over between 11 a.m. – 1 p.m. and dinner between 7 p.m. and 8 p.m. There must be six hours gap between lunch and dinner.
- Do not eat in a hurry. Chew and masticate food properly. Avoid cakes, cookies and fries.
- Wash hands with soap and water before every meal and after using the latrine.
- Maintain erect position while sitting or doing a desk job.
- Use unsaturated fats such as sunflower oil as cooking medium.
- Use steam cooked food; 50 per cent of meals should be salads.
- Eat one or two fruits before and after every meal.
- Avoid late dinner, heavy meals and late sleeping.
- Fast once every week with juice and water.
- Try to live on uncooked food at least once in a fortnight.
- Take enema when constipated and do *jalneti* regularly.
- Avoid smoking, alcohol, fried foods, white refined flour (maida) products, sugar, polished rice, flesh foods, junk foods, tea, coffee and cold drinks.
- Do not take cooked and raw things together.

- Live in a house that allows in adequate air and light.
- Do exercise, yoga, meditation regularly. Stay mobile and active, avoid sedentary lifestyle.
- Do not sacrifice the need for rest, relaxation and sleep at any cost. Leisure is pleasure. Take holidays. Spend time with nature.
- Depend on your body's natural healing power, vitalize it with disciplined life and balanced diet.
- Write down your thoughts, experiences, even if chaotic or off the cuff. It is the best way to calm your mind, reduce stress and boost your spirits.
- The fine art and science of living rests on six "H" pillars: Health, Home, Hygiene, Humanity, Harmony and Happiness.
- Prevent stress from becoming strain or distress. Only eight per cent of all our worries are "legitimate" cause for concern.
- Work in your areas of strength.
- We create our own mental, emotional, physical and spiritual environment by the attitude we develop.
- Avoid negative, vexatious people; they are a strain on your nerves.
- New studies have established the fact that people with deep spiritual commitments have better health and longer life.
- Forgiveness is a good medicine for angry vengeful thoughts. Forgive people and leave the past where it belongs.
- Think positive. Act positive. Be positive. ∎

FURTHER READINGS

1. Beth Ann Petro Roytal, *Sex Herbs*
2. Douglas J. Mason, *The Memory Workbook*
3. Acharya Mahaprajna, *Towards Inner Harmony*
4. John Ciancioni, *The Meditative Path*
5. Rechel Schaeffer, *Yoga for Your Spiritual Muscles*
6. Bernard Jensen, *Foods that Heal*
7. Cherie Calbom, *Juicing for Life*
8. N.N. Saha, *Raw Juice Therapy*
9. N.N. Saha, *Fruit & Vegetable Juice Therapy*
10. Ingfried Holeert, *Gauva: Medicine for Modern Diseases*
11. Herald W. Tietze, *Living food for Longer Life*
12. Robin Needes, *Naturopathy for Self-healing*
13. V.M. Kulkarni, *Healing through Naturopathy*
14. Worman Jollyman, *Good Health Naturally Without Drugs*

15. Michael A. Schmidt, *Beyond Antibiotics*

16. Ritu Arora, *Healthy Kitchen*

17. Aroona Reejhsinghani, *Feast on a Diabetic Diet*

18. R.P. Gupta, *Acupressure: Heal Yourself*

19. H.S. Khaneja, *Illustrated Guide to the Homoeopathic Treatment*

20. A.K. Mehta, *Health & Harmony through Ayurveda*

21. A.K. Bansal, *Magneto Therapy*

22. Jayce J. Morris, *Reiki: Hands that Heal*

Mail your order to

B. JAIN PUBLISHERS (P) LTD.
1921, Chuna Mandi, St. 10th Paharganj, New Delhi-110 055
Ph: 23580800, 51698991, 23581100, 23581300, 23583100
Fax: 011-23580471, 51698993; Email: bjain@vsnl.com
Website: www.bjainbooks.com